PRAISE FOR
"JUST A NURSE"

"A TIMELY AND ACCURATE PORTRAIT OF CONTEMPORARY AMERICAN NURSING. It is one of the most hopeful books I have read recently, illustrating how many nurses are working on ethical, economic, and social changes. The 2.5 million nurses in America are indeed a force for social good."

—Edward H. Halloran, R.N., Ph.D.,
Sr. Vice Pres./Director of Nursing,
University Hospitals of Cleveland

"INCISIVELY LAYS BARE A NURSE'S JOB—ITS REWARDS, ITS FRUSTRATIONS, ITS PROMISE, AS REPORTED BY NURSES THEMSELVES. IMPORTANT READING FOR ANYONE WHO HAS EVER BEEN A NURSE, OR WHO MAY EVER FACE BEING ILL IN OUR COUNTRY."

—Barbara Barnum, F.A.A.N.,
Editor, *Nursing and Health Care*

"CAPTURES THE SPIRIT OF NURSING. . . . This is a book for nurses and lay readers alike."

—Norma Lang, R.N., Ph.D., Dean and
Professor University of Wisconsin,
Milwaukee, School of Nursing

"THE INSIDER'S VIEWS HERE GIVE A HUMAN DIMENSION TO NURSING, dispel some of the mythology and stereotyping, and open appealing vistas for those considering nursing as a career."

—*Publishers Weekly*

"WONDERFUL READING . . . A LOVELY JOB IN SEARCHING OUT AND TOUCHING ON THE HEART OF THE AMERICAN NURSE."

—Echo Heron,
author of *Intensive Care*

JANET KRAEGEL, R.N., and
MARY KACHOYEANOS, R.N.

"JUST A NURSE"

From Clinic to Hospital Ward, Battleground to Cancer Unit—The Hearts and Minds of Nurses Today

A DELL BOOK

Published by
Dell Publishing
a division of
Bantam Doubleday Dell Publishing Group, Inc.
666 Fifth Avenue
New York, New York 10103

ISBN: 0-440-20763-0

Reprinted by arrangement with E. P. Dutton

Printed in the United States of America
Published simultaneously in Canada

September 1990

10 9 8 7 6 5 4 3 2 1

OPM

CONTENTS

FOREWORD

Without question we owe a debt of gratitude to all those who were trusting enough and selfless enough to let us disclose their innermost thoughts and poignant experiences. We thank them for their insights and their honesty. It was impossible to use all of the interviews; yet, we never left an interview without a new thought to pursue, a new perspective to be included in this book.

Everyone gave us a clearer vision of what nurses could be if they were truly valued, thereby offering us an additional incentive to describe their unique skills to the American public.

We used journalistic license in rearranging the nurses' words and sequence of thoughts. Because 97 percent of nurses are women, the pronoun *she* was used for nurse.

Interviews were gathered in many parts of the country. For the most part, names and places have been altered for obvious reasons.

We appreciate Tom Radlin, Ed Griffin, Ellie Fredericksen, Wilfred Kraegel, Marge Olszewski, Stefanie Tomescu, Jim Corona, Helen Kachoyeanos, David Black, and others for their constructive criticism.
A special thanks to Michael Schumacher for his assistance and belief in the inevitable publication of this book.

JANET M. KRAEGEL, R.N.
MARY K. KACHOYEANOS, R.N.

INTRODUCTION

Angels of mercy, mother figures, handmaidens, martinets, and sex symbols—these are the stereotypes of nurses depicted in romance novels, motion pictures, and prime-time television. We know nurses, however, who weep for their patients, save lives, fight the odds of their alcoholism, rant against doctors who treat them like morons, hatch the corporate business deals, go out on strike. Nurses are flesh-and-blood human beings who gripe, laugh, swear, sweat, dream, make mistakes, win and lose . . . just like everyone else.

It is time to bury nursing stereotypes, chip away the fantasies, and have nurses tell the public the truth about who they are, what they do, and what goes on in their heads and hearts.

People assume that a high caliber nurse will always be there when illness strikes. Not so! Enrollments in schools of nursing have fallen fifty percent in the last two years while enrollments of women in schools of medicine, law, and engineering have significantly increased. The catastrophic shortage of nurses affects every person who uses the health care system.

One solution proposed by the board of the American Medical Association is to train a registered care technologist (R.C.T.). The R.C.T.'s would be licensed to assume "a new role at the bedside" designed to "execute the medical protocols . . . with special emphasis on technical skills." As Sister Rosemary Donley, president of the National League for Nursing, aptly stated, "It is ironic and misguided that, at a time when patients require increasingly complex care, the AMA has decided we need lesser prepared practitioners at the bedside."

The independent decisions and actions of astute professional nurses make the difference between health and permanent disability, life or death. The nurse is the one who is in attendance in the dead of night when the executive with a coronary has a cardiac arrest. Nurses are the ones who will detect fetal distress during labor. When the hospital sends the patient home prematurely because his care is no longer reimbursed under DRGs it's the nurse who will go into the home and turn chaos into order.

As long as nurses have to bargain with others to attain control of their practice, the continuation of quality and competency in nursing care is in jeopardy.

There will always be someone who will be in attendance and do the technical tasks. Almost anyone can learn mechanical techniques. Whether these people will have the competency and commitment of most of the nurses described in this book will depend on all of us.

The public wants a nurse to be a warm, caring human being. The intellectual acumen needed to practice professional nursing is rarely understood. For instance, the image of Florence Nightingale is one of a mother figure bringing comfort to maimed soldiers. Few people know that Florence Nightingale was a renowned statistician who used epidemiological data to document the effectiveness of nursing practices. Because of her scientific analysis, disease and death were greatly reduced in the armies of the Crimea.

Since the days of Florence Nightingale, nurses have carried out medically delegated tasks. Nursing, however, represents a body of knowledge apart from medicine. The nurse, in carrying out nursing, also diagnoses and treats *human responses* to actual and potential health problems. Irrespective of the medical regimen, the nurse makes her own assessments as to how the patient and his or her family are adapting to the social and psychobiological effects of illness. In order to do this, the nurse establishes a reciprocal relationship with patient and family—and that can create magic. The patient, relieved of those burdens that impede physical progress, truly begins to heal.

The nurse's investment in other people's lives is not without a price. The patient or family member may reject her well-meaning efforts, or test her with hostility. Most of these relationships are meant to be transient. Investment of self leads to inevitable loss for the nurse. To deny herself these relationships through unwillingness to invest in others—or through contempt or indifference—is to miss the essence of nursing.

How the nurse responds to the patient's needs will depend on her level of education, experience, commitment, and the time afforded her to do her nursing. The nurses who reveal themselves in this book have the education, experience, and commitment. They discuss the problems they have finding time to practice nursing in today's health care system.

The first step in any social crisis is to raise the public's awareness of what is happening and why. This book is a series of interviews with practicing nurses throughout the country. As they explain their daily work situations, the underlying reasons for the nursing crisis become apparent. The voices of these nurses illuminate the deepest crevices and the highest pinnacles of the profession.

Certainly there are nurses who enter the profession inspired by visions of alleviating human suffering, but there are others who got washed into the profession on a wave of last resort. Certainly nurses can be found racing down busy hospital corridors, hands filled with complex apparatus, but the majority of real nursing is the use of *self* in monitoring, assessing, guiding, teaching, nurturing, supporting, and counseling patients. Nursing has a code that expresses the value system of the profession, and these interviews show how nurses interpret that code in their practice.

Nurses' human failings are acknowledged in this book. Conversations with frustrated, chemically dependent, and disenchanted nurses poignantly speak of the human limits of physical stamina and psychological strength. Hard, unromantic facts are interwoven with dammed-up hurts and glowing satisfactions. The unfolding of the hectic lives of these modern-day nurses creates the colorful, fascinating mosaic of a vast, unsettled profession.

Even today, bright young people are frequently discouraged by their high school counselors and families from being "just a nurse." As one of the nurses interviewed put it, "My father said that all a nurse needs is a strong back and weak mind." What emerges from these interviews is a conviction that nursing requires a strong back, a keen mind, and a very strong will. This book describes all that being "just a nurse" implies.

JANET KRAEGEL, R.M.
MARY KACHOYEANOS, R.M.

PART ONE

BEING THERE

Care of patients is a constant, twenty-four-hour-a-day process, and responsibility for that process rests squarely on the shoulders of the professional nurse. Being there, over time, she becomes sensitive to patients' physical changes and unspoken words—a wince of pain, a dry cough, untouched food, a change in the color of the drainage on the dressing.

The nurse weighs, sifts, organizes, or charts these clues. She decides whether a clue is irrelevant or significant, whether it bears watching or calls for her immediate response.

Being there over time allows a relationship to develop between the nurse, the patient, the patient's family. The touching, the listening, the alertness to what is said create an atmosphere of personal trust that can lead to a patient sharing confidences not easily disclosed to others.

When the sun goes down, anxieties go up. Patients' fears, worry, uncertainty, and feelings of abandonment are altered when nurses are there to listen and insightfully respond.

1

Beth—The Burn Nurse

Care of burn patients is tough: Rarely can nurses endure the exposure—day after day, year after year—to the excruciating physical and emotional pain of burn patients. Beth is an exception. She has "worked burns" since 1969.

When I came here for a tour prior to nursing school, they took us through the burn unit. I almost didn't go into nursing after that. As students, we rotated to burns and I got hooked, I guess, because I felt I'd be able to do so much good for people.

Last weekend I split shifts with another nurse and worked from seven A.M. to seven P.M. I thought, "Oh, God, I can't do this." I was worn out and my feet were killing me. Nursing is a young woman's profession.

I've stayed on the burn unit this long because of the strong working relationships we nurses have. When we're mad, we let it out among ourselves. If the strain of taking care of an especially severe burn patient gets to be too much, we relieve each other. We just know, from the nurse's behavior, that continually being in there with that patient is getting to be too much.

We work directly with the attending physicians. They are great to work with, but they expect too much. They whip in and out, leaving us to monitor the patients' charts and tell them when the electrolytes are off or the blood count's up. That's their job, not ours. They forget that.

One time, a doctor had a grafting set for a Monday. It was to be on a guy's leg only, but after I had the patient in the tub, I could see some other areas on the arms that also needed grafts. I called the doctor on a Saturday at his lake house and told him. He said, "OK, I'll look at them when I get back." Sure enough, he grafted the arms, too.

I get sort of mad about this. Don't get me wrong—this doctor is terrific, but *he's* the one being paid to medically assess the patient, not me. We nurses are well-equipped to recognize when grafts are needed, and we know enough to prescribe treatments, but these kinds of decisions are the doctor's responsibility. If the doctor is too busy, we should be legally allowed to do some of this and get paid for it.

We once treated a young guy named Jeff. Boy, he was a good-looking son-of-a-gun. He had been tarring a roof when he fell into the scalding tar. His scalp, ears, and back were burned—about fifty percent of his body, in all. I still remember his screams during the daily treatments. We'd place him in a Hubbard tank with the water swirling, then scrub him with rough gauze four-by-fours to scrape off the dead skin. Hours of cleansings, graftings, and dressings went into his care. God, we'd all be exhausted.

When he was finally on his way to recovery, he went into a depression. This happens a lot. You never know why, or when, it will happen, but you always prepare to be there, to be available.

One night, I went into Jeff's room and just sat at his bedside a few minutes. His behavior had changed recently, so I said, "If you want to talk about something, I'm here."

He was looking straight ahead, not wanting eye-to-eye contact. Tears started to roll down his cheeks. That's always hard—especially for a big, macho guy. I guess he needed a mother figure for a nurse, because he spilled his guts to me. It turned out that a few days before, he had dropped his newspaper and, because his back was healing, he couldn't bend over to pick it up. Just like that, it all came to a head. He felt like he'd never be a real man again, or work in construction.

But that wasn't all. His relationship with his wife was in trouble. I'd gotten to know her really well. They were from a small town upstate. They had two small kids and little money, so my roommate and I let them stay in our apartment when they came down to visit on weekends. Apparently, Jeff had fooled around quite a bit, but his wife loved him and just ignored it. Jeff brought a lot of their problems to his burn situation: He needed to find out if his wife still loved him, and he needed to know if he would always be a macho man to her, even if his good looks were gone and other girls no longer found him attractive. I persuaded them to get some counseling.

We do a great deal of patient and family teaching. I used to go out and do follow-up home visits, too. We found that patients could be discharged earlier if a nurse could follow-up with them. That was fine for a while, but I was spending too much extra time at work and not enough time at home. I now have a family and small kids, so I've quit that and only work half-time. Frankly, that's enough.

We keep in touch with lots of our patients, and we have former burn patients coming back to visit all the time. One woman, who had lost her kids in a house fire, was with us for six months. After she went to the rehabilitation hospital, I would visit her and bring my little girl along. That seemed to help her. Now she comes back here as a volunteer, to talk to other patients. This unit depends on patients and former patients helping each other out.

Nurses can tell patients about the really frightening realities of getting burned, and we try to reassure them that their symptoms will go away, but it's hard for them to believe us. It's so much better for a former patient, who has experienced the same thing, to tell a new patient of the realities. It's more believable when he hears it from a soul partner that made it through.

Volunteers and patients become very close to each other, and to us. As a matter of fact, I met my husband in the unit—he'd been a patient and three years later he looked me up again. We hit it off and got married eight years ago.

We've had patients we couldn't help, like the mother

whose small kids died in a house fire last winter. She was badly burned, but she recovered enough to go home, and then she killed herself. Then there was a gal who was in here with burns from attempted suicide. She did the same thing: We got her well—whatever that means—and she went home and hanged herself.

Do you remember the story of the husband who set fire to his wife after he'd watched the TV movie *The Burning Bed*? The woman was estranged from her husband, and he hid at her place until she came home one evening, and then he poured gasoline on her and set her on fire. He turned her into a human torch. The flames scorched her entire body except for the soles of her feet.

We took care of her here. There was no question that she was going to die. She was told, as was her family. It was terrible for her. When the fluid in her lungs got too great, she had to have a tube put down her throat to her lungs. She couldn't talk, and she could only communicate with her eyes. Finally, the swelling shut her eyelids, and she went into a coma. The skin she had left looked like parchment, brown and black and thickened. The skin died, and it was like taking care of a living corpse.

We turned her hourly, gave her pain medications, and saw that her family was cared for. She smelled horrible from the rotting skin. It was emotionally hard for us to take care of her. The family, too, could hardly stay in the room. Mercifully, she died in a week but, you know, when I get to heaven I'm going to ask God why it was necessary. Why did she even have to suffer that whole week?

2

A Gift to Be Human

Ricky's career has been exclusively in oncology nursing, beginning ten years ago at the National Cancer Institute. She is now a clinical specialist in a large catchment area for AIDS patients in New York City.

I don't know life without AIDS. It's part of every nurse's practice, whether you're in pediatrics, obstetrics, psychiatry, or here. You'll always be dealing with AIDS. Our hospital borders a highly gay community, and we have a special AIDS in-patient unit. Between that unit and the AIDS patients on the cancer unit, we average about fifty-five AIDS in-patients per day.

When I first started working here, there weren't that many AIDS patients. Because my specialty is oncology, I'd seen most of the AIDS patients who presented with some type of neoplastic condition, such as lymphoma or Kaposi's sarcoma. Over the years, AIDS has become a specialty.

When the idea of an AIDS unit was first proposed, we all said, "Oh, my God! Who'd want to work there?" But nurses do. They all volunteered to work there. They have physician support, too. They're all learning together. It's a very exciting thing, because they're the forerunners. If there's a question about AIDS, they're the people you ask. For nursing, that's a plus. You are seen as an expert. It helps in retention, both on the AIDS unit and on the oncology unit.

People with cancer and AIDS needs good physical care. They need body massage, cleansing, care of bedsores, oral hygiene, and pain medications. They need someone who will do these things with sincerity and not be repulsed by the look of a rotting, wasting body. All the nurses on the AIDS unit are very care-oriented. I walked on the unit once and a nurse was dancing in the hall with a patient.

We also have a supportive care program that deals with AIDS patients who are dying in the home. It's one of the few in the country. The supportive care program is similar to a hospice program. The team consists of nurses, social workers, and volunteers. The nurses do hands-on work and psychosocial tasks such as counseling and planning funerals. Not too long ago, there was only one funeral home in the area that would bury a person who died from AIDS. Nurses and social workers had to find places that would bury these people. It's not as much of a problem in New York City, but it still exists. In fact, I recently gave a talk in a neighboring city on Long Island. It was like going into a different world. We're so used to AIDS here that we forget the prejudices and unwarranted fears. The supportive care unit is there for the patient and family. It's a very necessary component of the care of patients and their families.

I'm not going to say that, just because we're in a large catchment area, there's no fear—there is. And I think the fear is justified. It's fear of getting stuck with an infected needle, no matter how careful you are. Right now, we're looking at our I.V. policy. We're cutting down the number of steps, because each step brings greater chance of getting stuck. We don't recap our needles anymore. We toss them into a thick plastic container. The disease has made us all look at what we do. We wear gloves when we're in contact with blood or excrement. Masks and gloves are recommended if you are doing any procedure in which there might be some splatter, or when patients are on respiratory precautions. Very few patients are in isolation here. We don't consider them to be lepers, although some places still do.

Many patients coming into the hospital are frightened about acquiring AIDS through blood transfusions. Actually, their fears are unwarranted. We've become painfully aware of the route of transmission, and we have the best screening techniques in the country. Actually, the patient paranoia has decreased. It's a matter of common sense.

Our patients are from all walks of life. They're I.V. drug abusers, bisexual married people, homosexuals, those who have acquired the disease by contaminated blood transfusions—the gamut. My practice, by necessity, has become limited. I see only those AIDS patients with lymphoma, which is one of the types of cancers that AIDS patients can get. It's systemic and very debilitating. These patients are on multiple types of chemotherapy—some as many as six to eight drugs at a time.

They have the concerns any patient with cancer has. Unlike some other types of cancer, AIDS is life-limiting. It hurts to see people your own age dying. At first, you wonder why they go through all the pain of therapy. Sure, for other patients with lymphoma, you'd say, "Go for it!" Most likely, they'll be cured or have a long remission. Not so with AIDS. Most of them are survivors; they want to live. They'll think, "If you can take care of my lymphoma, maybe I'll make it until the miracle drug is found."

Most of our patients die of infections or viruses. We have all age groups. We don't have children here, and I'm glad for that. The youngest I've seen was eighteen. Our patients are very stratified, too. The homosexual population seems to be more sophisticated, more attuned to their disease, than are the I.V. drug users. That's an obvious socioeconomic fact, with or without the disease. So, in some ways, it's easier to deal with the homosexuals, because they're very intelligent, very motivated, and will stick to the treatment regimen. A lot of these people will want this treatment at home. They'll want to spend as much time at home as possible. They have tremendous support systems.

AIDS patients can be very hard patients to care for. When the virus goes to their brains, they have mental status changes. When they get dementia, which can be permanent, you need to find someone to stay with them. Right now, with the nursing shortage, that's difficult. Sometimes we get their lovers or volunteers or nurse's aides to sit with them.

The majority of care is nursing. Like other cancers, after the surgery, after the chemo and radiation, it's nursing that the patient needs. It's the bridge that makes the difference between discomfort and comfort.

The nurse does a total assessment. She knows to set up mouth care and get the humidifier, because the patient's secretions are thick and obstruct their breathing. If the patient is having uncontrollable diarrhea, it is the nurse who is in there looking at the skin, attending to skin care, getting an air mattress. The nurse is the one who is assessing the patient's nutritional status. She is the one who gets the special food or recruits a family member to do so. It's the nurse who's there when the patient is upset and crying, especially on those long, dark nights. It's also the nurse who develops a day-to-day rapport with the patient. Patients can feel comfortable sharing their physical and emotional pain. There is a lot of intimacy involved; it's the same intimacy found with anyone who is terminal. For some reason, people who are dying tend to lessen their barriers. It's a sad phenomenon that we wait until that time to establish those relationships. But it's a privilege for nurses to work in this area, because in no other type of work are you invited into another's soul, so to speak. That's a special gift.

We had a young AIDS patient who was in and out until he died two Thanksgivings ago. We knew more about him when he died than a lot of people probably know about their own families or friends. We got to know his whole family, and we knew that he'd been in the Peace Corps. His family brought in photo albums, which were a reflection of his life and what he looked like before the disease ravaged him. He shared his journals, and his favorite music, with us.

We went through the illness with the family. We shared their optimism and then their resignation when it became obvious that he could not lick the disease. Yes, it was horrible that they lost this twenty-eight-year-old, but together we all got through it. They shared their vulnerability and fears with us, and we nurses also shared our fears, our vulnerability, with them.

When he was dying, he had a lot of nasal bleeding. The only way to stop it was nasal packing, which was extremely uncomfortable and made it difficult for him to breathe. We all felt terrible being unable to ease his discomfort. We huddled in the hall with the family, trying to figure out what we could do to make it better for him. We can't always win, but people know we try, we care. We keep fighting, keep trying. Sometimes we win, and sometimes we lose. The important thing is people know we don't give up.

People react differently to the diagnosis. It depends on the person. We see people who initially try therapy and then say, "Thank you very much, I've tried therapy and it's not working." They'll take their money out of the bank and go off to Europe. Then there are the others, who wait until the end for the miracle cure. It's really like a response to any other terminal illness.

I've never had a homosexual patient say, "My God, if I hadn't practiced this lifestyle I wouldn't be in this fix." Nor have I heard an I.V. drug user berate himself. I don't know about the people who got AIDS from contaminated blood transfusions; I imagine they feel differently. It would make an interesting study. By the time we see AIDS patients, it no longer matters how they got the disease. Bitterness doesn't last that long; sadness takes over. It's funny, too, because we have married couples with the disease, and they don't dissipate energy on the "whys"; they use their energy to fight the disease.

The gays are angry that the disease has hit their "group," and angry because they believe the government is holding back on finding a cure. In some ways, that's what's made them so cohesive and so political. It's probably why the research effort has been so strong.

I like to get new things going and then move on. I've set up new units, and I've done staff and patient education. Right now, I'm involved in setting up an out-patient AIDS unit. I also have a grant to teach breast self-exams in the city.

I just enrolled in a course on reflexology and massage therapy to use with my patients. My dream is to set up a spa-type "wellness center" for cancer patients. I don't believe hospitals are the place to look at both health and wellness. At best, you leave a hospital on the same level you were on before you got ill. If we want to make people healthier, we need to explore more avenues. In oncology, we've been using drugs, surgery, and radiation, and though they kill the cancer, they take their toll. Though I believe in these therapies, I also believe we could use other therapies as adjuncts. Surgery often disfigures patients and causes body-image problems. I've found that body massage, imaging, helps people to reestablish their body boundaries and makes them feel better about themselves.

I'm currently working with a woman who is hospitalized and in the terminal phase of her cancer. She's fairly immobilized. I use body massage, rubbing her back and extremities. By the time I'm done, she is relaxed enough to sleep undisturbed for several hours. That's a real therapy. We can use a combination of the Eastern therapies, meditation, massage, and relaxation to help people be the best they can be at that point in time. If you are relaxed, your body will react differently. It isn't going to cure your cancer, but it will make you feel better and perhaps more receptive to the therapy. I actually have a place to do outpatient therapy. We're going to set it up shortly. It's interesting—a couple of surgeons and nurses are very interested in the idea.

Sure, we're all frightened at times. My sister is an OB-GYN practitioner. She worked with a large Haitian population in Florida, and they screened all their patients. When she transferred to Boston, she was totally shocked to find that she needed legal consent to screen patients. She was really upset when she was called in to do a vaginal exam on a psychiatric patient who'd been an I.V. drug abuser. She was told she couldn't get a titer [blood test for AIDS] on the patient unless she had the patient's legal consent. That poses problems for practitioners treating those patients. They really have a right to know who they're dealing with, but right now the law doesn't provide them that access.

It's ironic—patients are constantly thanking us for whatever we are doing. What they don't realize is they are giving us a gift by allowing us to be human. They give us the opportunity to share who we are, which is something we don't get to do in everyday life. It's an intimacy that would never happen in other situations. I think nurses are privileged. We get to share that more than any other group in health care—or anywhere else, for that matter. I think it's because we are the hands-on people. We have been physically intimate with people in terms of their bodily functions. We're also emotionally intimate. Over time, you naturally share a part of yourself.

3

The Beat Goes On

Janet works in a cardiac care unit (CCU) of a hospital. She has come in to see us during her off-hours to discuss her practice with cardiac patients.

All of our patients have had some type of heart attack. I decide what they need to know to get through this experience and avoid coming back with another heart attack.

I got hooked on coronary care mainly due to the influence of a specialist nurse. I saw her practice on the CCU when I was a senior student. She was a dynamo who knew coronary care inside out. Just by looking at a patient, she intuitively knew if he was likely to arrest.

At first I wasn't confident enough to take the responsibility of working in such an intense environment. After graduation, I took a job as the only camp nurse for over five hundred developmentally-delayed adults and children. I figured that if I could handle that responsibility, I could manage coronary care patients. That was over four years ago.

When I first started working there, I took a hard look at our critical care unit. It was really buzzing. The monitors were chugging out the pictures of the patients' heart rates. The nurses were busy checking vital signs. I thought, "We're doing a lot of service here. We're paying a lot of attention to the body, but little to the person."

I did a lot of reading about sudden death. The suggestions were to talk to the comatose patients, even though you think they don't hear you. Sometimes, during a code [a cardiac arrest], it's all you can do to get the physical things done. But even when cardiac arrest occurs and I'm at the head of the bed, bagging the person [giving respiratory aid], I'll talk to the patient. I'll say something like, "Mr. Clark, it's OK, we're here to help you. You'll feel us pressing on your chest. You're getting medication in your I.V." At first, the staff looked at me as though I'd cracked. Now they're used to me.

What good does it do? I can't tell you. Usually, people who make it through a code can't recall being spoken to. Most of their recollections are of lights and tunnels—the typical descriptions you've heard when people describe having come back from the dead. I remember one lady who asked me, "Why'd you bring me back? It was so peaceful there." It sort of gives you the chills.

CCU involves so much high tech. I noticed how uncomfortable patients are in the midst of all those machines, and I wondered what we could do to increase their comfort. I began rubbing patients' backs, and I noticed that they seemed to relax. Some got drowsy. For years, nurses rubbed backs to provide a source of comfort for patients; lately, however, the back rub hasn't been used. I asked myself how therapeutic the back rub was to patients. I began to study it, collect data. Since patients are on monitors, I could see on the screen that the back rub was decreasing the work of their hearts.

Some things I do to provide quality care cannot be measured. For instance, if the patient is comatose, I focus on the family. What place does the family want in the person's dying? Do they want to be with him? Talk to him? Some people can do this very easily; for others, it's too much to ask.

I recall a patient who had been admitted with sudden death, had been revived, and was comatose. One day, he appeared to be more alert. When his wife entered the unit, I said to him, "Mr. Blake, give your wife a kiss." I'll be damned if he didn't rise up and do just that. He never again regained consciousness.

His wife and I had formed a close attachment. A few months after his death, she called me. She said everything had settled now, that things were going well, and she wanted to thank me for helping her through her husband's death. She said, "I don't miss him too much because I have him here." It took a minute for me to realize that she'd had him cremated and placed in an urn.

Recently, I was in a restaurant where his daughter also happened to be dining. She beckoned me to her table and introduced me to her friends. She told everybody, "This is the nurse who helped Daddy die peacefully." It was nice to know people appreciated and remembered you.

Some nurses are uncomfortable dealing with the family of a patient who is dying. It isn't that they don't know how —they've had enough in-service training to learn the skills. I've seen nurses simply hand the bereaved person a card and say, "Here's the name of the funeral home; call them when you get home." I try to make the phone calls for them. I stay close. If there's no other family present, I see that the spouse gets home safely.

Then there's the case of a lady in her late forties who was admitted with chest pain last winter. Naturally, she was frightened. The doctor told her, "If the pain continues, you'll need a cardiac catheterization tomorrow—possibly open-heart surgery." Well, how many people would admit to pain, given that prognosis? The lady was a wreck.

I was concerned that she'd deny her pain. It was the holiday season, and the biggest thing on her mind was to be home for Christmas. I sat at her bedside and said, "Look, Brenda, I know you want to be home for Christmas. Denying your pain won't get you there. If the reason for your pain can be diagnosed, chances are you'll get home faster. Tell me when you have pain." She answered that she would.

A while later, she pulled her call light on. I answered it. She told me she was having pain. She said, "Whatever they do, please don't let them take me up without seeing my boys first." I promised that I wouldn't. The next morning, the two boys came early to see their mother.

During the catheterization, her heart arrested. They had to shock her several times to get her heart started again. When the doctor came to give her the catheterization results, he cryptically told her, "We found some blockage. We're transferring you to Mountain Valley Hospital in the morning for an angioplasty. Frankly, I don't think it will work. I predict you'll need a by-pass."

I was in a dilemma. I didn't want to add to her anxiety, but she needed to know what to expect, should surgery become a reality. I sat down and described the procedure. I told her what intensive care would be like. She said, "You told me nothing was going to happen yesterday, and I almost died. Now I'm in for more risk. What makes you think it won't happen again?"

I understood her mistrust. I said, "I can't tell you that nothing will happen; it certainly is always a possibility. Remember, though, that you are essentially healthy. The odds are in your favor that things will go well." She had the angioplasty and didn't require the by-pass surgery. It's always a struggle, deciding how far to stick your neck out.

A lot of learning goes on continually between the resident physicians and the nurses. The residents don't resent this; they depend on the nurses to know the particular protocol of an attending physician. Physicians have individual drug preferences, even though they're treating the same thing. It takes time to learn the individual physician's likes and dislikes. The resident counts on us to clue him in. You find yourself directing the resident on the medical treatment for a very sick person. That's sort of scary.

It's our responsibility to call the patient's physician if we think the resident physician is using poor judgment. For example, we may determine that the patient is retaining too much water, or that his color is poor. If the resident doesn't take action, even though he's supposed to be the link to the cardiologist, I'll call the physician directly. I won't wait. The attending physicians trust our judgment and expect us to alert them.

We also stick our necks out when codes are called. Most

times, we are the first to respond when the patient codes. We have a system between ICU, coronary care, and the step-down unit so we can respond, as a team, to any code. We start the procedures to resuscitate, start I.V.'s, and get the patient hooked up to the monitor. We give lidocaine, atropine, and shock the patient. Usually, by this time, the resident on call takes over. If not, we go ahead and do it all. Until new residents have sufficient experience, the nurses usually run the scene.

The other day I ran to a code on the step-down unit. Two nurses and the resident were working on the patient. One nurse was bagging the patient and coaching the doctor along, asking, "Does the patient have a pulse? Are you going to give the epinephrine now?" The nurse was the one to take control. You need to have a lot of experience before you can function quickly. Residents have to get the experience.

The nurse even directed the doctor on where to place the needle in a pericardial tap. I didn't think that was right. She'd never done one either. We're not allowed to perform those procedures. She had seen one; he hadn't seen any. The resident followed the nurse's direction. Fortunately, it worked out okay.

It is flattering to think that the doctor uses your assessments in deciding on his care, but it's disturbing, too. Frequently, you'll see these fellows taking what you've written in your work-up of the patient and transferring the comments verbatim into their history and physicals. I get nervous with that. In the eighties, there's no place for people who can't cut the mustard—doctors or nurses.

I like to see the patients when they come back for their clinic visits in outpatient. I also make a point to attend the monthly Heart Beat meetings for discharged patients. The group meets for support and additional teaching. They enjoy seeing their nurses, and we enjoy seeing them doing well. It keeps a link.

Unfortunately, some come back to CCU with another attack. Most of these people are older patients who never could tolerate surgery. They may be back with heart attacks two or three times before they die. The good thing is that the two or three years of added life had an extra quality for them. They knew their days were numbered, so they made the most of their time.

4

Suffer the Little Children

Jayne coordinates a bone marrow transplant program for children. She takes us to the transplant unit, where all the children are in private rooms, isolated from the lethal germs of the outside world. We look through the glass window in the door to the room of a one-year-old. The baby, attached to several monitors and other life-saving paraphernalia, seems oblivious of us. He lies in a fetal position.

Sure, caring for dying kids can be *very* depressing. You look for the little gains, such as the kids who survive through the next year. I stay in this business because of the kids—they keep me going. The other day, I sat down with a little five-year-old, who showed me a picture he'd drawn. He said it was a picture of a hospital. The exits from the hospital were at the top of the building, and at the bottom he'd drawn a door. He said, "When you enter here, you don't return." He was telling me exactly how he was feeling. He'd been through three operations and was at the end-stage of his disease. The last try was to be a bone marrow transplant. He was able to share his fears with me, and I was able to help reassure him and make him feel a little better. It's a two-way street in this business.

Since I was in nursing school, I knew that I had something special to offer these kids, that I could make a difference, and that's where I've devoted my career. Before I came here, I worked in a general cancer program for children. I liked that. Though everyone was aware of the child's total needs, we all took different roles. The physician concentrated on the medical needs of the child; he determined what drugs were needed and how the child was physically responding to the disease. I did all the teaching. I told the children—at their level of understanding—and their parents what would happen, how the drugs would work. I administered all the chemotherapeutic drugs and stayed with those kids to the end, whether the end was cure and life, or death. It was good that I could start with the child and parent early in the disease because they learned how to deal with the psychosocial implications as well as how to deal with the effects of the drugs.

Parents needed to know how a disease would change their child's life—how it would change the family and how they could manage—so it wasn't so devastating. The child needed help, too, so the disease wouldn't become overwhelming and distort his life. That's where I made the difference.

The physician I worked with didn't have the time to spend with families, but I did. I liked that job very much, because the children and their parents were tied to me, so to speak. I was the one they called when they needed answers.

For example, there was little Bruce, who'd been born with congenital leukemia. He'd been disease-free for several years. Then, at the age of six, his symptoms reappeared. That relapse was as devastating to the family as it had been the first time around.

The physician was rather matter-of-fact in his assessment. "These are your chances. We'll try this course of chemotherapy. If that doesn't work, we'll try another." Well, that's realistic, but it doesn't help people get through the illness.

Bruce was very aware of the possibility that he might die. He talked about it with me and drew pictures that were even more telling than his words. His mother and I became very close. We'd talk a lot. She wanted factual information, but even more, she wanted someone to listen to her, someone who cared. It meant a lot to me when the mother wrote to me, after Bruce had died, and said, "Jayne, I'll never forget you; you made such a difference in our lives." It's been several years, and I still hear from her and from other families.

I try to protect myself emotionally, because it does hurt too much. I was twenty-one when I first cared for a child dying of cancer. I remember him turning his face on the pillow, looking at me with those large eyes and saying, "Bye." Five minutes later, this five-year-old was dead. That's hard—it breaks your heart. I went to his funeral. I don't go to many funerals now. . . . I say good-bye at another point, like when the child goes home or when he dies in the hospital. I don't like funerals.

After I left my job in another state, eight kids died within six months. The parents wrote to let me know the kids had died. I wrote back, but I was sort of relieved that I wasn't there when the kids died.

The hardest thing is telling the other kids that one of their peers has died. These kids get very attached to each other. I had to tell a sixteen-year-old that another teenager, who was in therapy with her, had died. It wasn't easy. I started out by saying, "Peggy, I have something sad to tell you." She was stunned. She was grieving the death of her friend, but she was also concerned for herself. We talked about why Tara had died, and how her progression was different from Peggy's disease. We talked about the fact that Tara had been in great pain and how she now was at peace. Peggy was very religious, so we talked about Tara's being in heaven with Jesus, though I wouldn't say something like that if the family wasn't religious.

Sometimes, the kids ask, "Am I going to die?" I always start out by asking them why they are asking that. Why are they concerned that they are going to die now? I tell them I know that, when they are not feeling well, they are scared they may die. I try to help them see that they're not as sick as the child who died.

Of course, some kids are. Then you need to deal with what the parents want. Not too many kids ask me that. They seem to be protective of the adults. I've had parents who wanted to keep the diagnosis of cancer from the child. It's unrealistic, especially when a child is a teenager. Even the younger kids know they are very sick. I talk with the parents about their fears. Sometimes, they feel more secure and can tell the child and act like they know the disease will be licked.

These kids go through a lot. Lots of times, the kids will tell me, "Jayne, I don't want to do this anymore." We talk about how tough it is. It isn't pleasant—the discomfort and pain from the treatments, the nausea and the vomiting. We are constantly looking for ways to make things a little easier on them. The kids with leukemia have several bone marrow aspirations and spinal taps during the course of their disease. My colleagues and I are doing a study using self-relaxation techniques and play therapy. We also teach the kids ways to cope with the procedures, such as using breathing exercises, imagery, and a sort of self-hypnosis. These kids go through these procedures better than some adults.

We're just starting bone marrow transplantation. It's alternative therapy for those who want it. It can cure the child. It does entail a lot of suffering very similar to aggressive chemotherapy. The kids are uncomfortable for a long time. They have trouble with mouth sores. Some have severe, persistent diarrhea. They generally feel bad. Our biggest concern is massive infections. But if the graft takes and you can get them through all the other things, the disease is usually licked.

One thing that's hard for people to understand is that, once the decision is made to transplant the child, we don't give up until the bitter end. We all fight hard for that patient. We've made a commitment to that child and family to do all in our power to get him through. We'll put the child on a ventilator if need be. People wonder why we're going to such lengths. It's a different philosophy. We leave the decision to the parents.

Then you have the physician who doesn't believe in transplant. When his patient no longer responds to traditional therapy, he decides to refer for transplant. Unfortunately, it's too late. The child cannot respond to therapy, so we refuse to transplant. That's hard for the physician, too, because he's very attached to his patients and wants to do everything in his power to cure them.

One of the first kids I saw here was a thirteen-year-old who could have benefited from a transplant. Her physician was against it, so she didn't have the transplant. I was very angry about Myra's death because I'm still convinced she would be alive today if she'd had a transplant. I tried to intervene. I wrote letters to her parents, telling them about the transplant option, hoping they'd write and ask about it. But they never did. Who knows? Maybe they couldn't face it. Maybe they couldn't afford it.

Myra wrote to me two weeks before she relapsed. I still have that letter. She was so excited. She was coming off chemotherapy, her arterial line was out, her hair was growing back. Life was rosy. Two weeks later, I got a call saying she had relapsed.

As a transplant coordinator, I get calls from physicians, and I collect all the information needed to determine if the child is an active candidate for transplant. The information is then evaluated at a team conference, and then either I or the head physician will discuss the child's candidacy with the referring physician.

Once the child enters our system, I do all the appropriate preparation and teaching of the child and parents. I lay out the options for them. The parents then decide whether to transplant or not. We tell them everything that will or could happen, but people don't really hear the bad stuff until it happens. I guess it's a defense mechanism.

Parents want to do everything possible to save their child's life. They'll insist on a transplant when it's clear that the child will not benefit. Then you have to tell them, "No, we're sorry, your child isn't a candidate for a transplant." That's tough to do. The other factor is that, in a day of research, the medical community looks for results. They don't want to do transplants in which the patients die, so they aren't willing to chance it if the child is a poor candidate.

That sounds cruel, but it really protects the kids. Why put a child through all that misery, when you're almost certain that he hasn't a chance of recovery? That would be really cruel. At first, not going to the nth degree was hard for me, but when I think of a child dying a gruesome death, I see how much better off he is dying peacefully with his family. In this business, you finally come to terms with death. We can't cure everyone, but we can make it easier for them as they're dying. What makes it all worthwhile is a smile from a child who is cured.

5

A Certain Kind of Caring

Jody sandwiches our conversation between her kids' lunch break from school and her graduate class at a local university. Her beagle snuggles at her feet as she recounts her thirteen years' experience as an obstetrical nurse.

My mother became ill when I was in pre-med school. I was surprised to find the family was given only a few minutes of the physician's time, whereas the nurses were with us constantly, watching and reassuring. It was a nurse who monitored my mother's condition and called the physician when my mother took a turn for the worse. She saved her life—really.

When the time came for me to make a conscious career decision, I decided that I wanted that kind of patient contact, so I chose nursing. It's a decision I've never regretted.

When I completed nursing school, I married and moved to a small town in the northern part of the state. Nurses with baccalaureate degrees were scarce up there. After a few months, I was offered the pick of two managerial positions. Since I lacked management experience, I declined the offers and opted for a staff position in obstetrics.

I stayed there for three years. The rural environment provided experiences I'd never find in the big city. It wasn't unusual to see a woman delivering her thirteenth child. I alone delivered over one hundred babies during that time. The doctor may have been only five minutes away, but the baby was only two minutes away.

My first solo delivery was precipitous. The doctor had checked the lady and told me that she had a way to go. He left to make rounds in another part of the hospital. He was no sooner gone when the mother said, "The baby is coming." I said, "It can't be. The doctor said you're nowhere ready to deliver." She answered, "I don't care what he said. It's coming."

Sure enough, there was the brow of the head. Since it was a brow presentation, the doctor had felt the soft spot of the baby's head instead of the woman's cervix.

When the doctor returned, the lady had delivered—in the labor room. He chastised me for not having gotten her into the delivery room. The patient stood up for me. She said, "You're the one who told her I wasn't ready." After that, I learned to trust the moms above anyone else. A lady delivering her thirteenth kid is usually right.

Right from the beginning, I liked maternal-child nursing. I liked being part of the changes in maternity nursing. During the early seventies, we started childbirth classes for couples, and it has now become full-blown family-centered maternity care.

The seventies were years of contrasts. Some moms wanted husband participation and wanted to be awake during delivery, while others wanted to be by themselves and asleep. Couples fought to control the deliveries in their own ways. We were constantly trying to accommodate their needs by putting our own values on the back burner.

When we moved to the city, I became very active in the natural childbirth movement. I'm particularly committed to the idea of consumers' being decision makers. I'm disturbed that we're losing ground in consumer advocacy. Today's consumers are limited in the options for childbirth available to them.

People used to come to childbirth classes to learn about childbirth options such as Lamaze, midwifery, or the Reed method. We didn't push any particular way to have a baby. We'd list the pros and cons, and they'd decide on the type of birth they wanted. Now, hospitals are capturing patients by marketing their childbirth classes. The options presented are limited by the philosophy of the physicians on the hospital's staff. With HMOs [Health Maintenance Organizations], people are locked into a particular hospital, and feel they must go along with the preferences of that hospital's physician. The options are really still available, but the women aren't choosing them as often as they used to.

Nor are women as oriented to free choices as they were a few years ago. People aren't saying, "I want to do it my way." Previously, a woman would walk in and say, "I don't want monitoring. I don't want I.V's. I want to have my child in a birthing chair." Today, women are saying, "Whatever the physician wants is okay with me."

Surprisingly, the newer breed of male physician is less consumer-oriented than the older male physicians and women physicians. The older doctor says, "No matter what the rule says, if the mother wants an additional person in the delivery room, then that's what she'll have." The younger guy says, "The rule says only one support person can be with the woman in labor. That's it. No exceptions." The younger physician epitomizes omnipotence. He wants control. He uses everything he was taught: fetal monitors, I.V's, anesthesia—the works.

Patients who are seen by physician groups in HMOs can run up against real conflicts. Take the case we had last week. Ms. Duchek and her primary physician, Dr. Worley, had agreed on intermittent monitoring. Dr. Worley wasn't available when she went into labor. The on-call physician insisted on continuous monitoring, so there was Ms. Duchek, stuck with continuous monitoring.

When the on-call doctor orders fetal monitoring, the nurse is legally bound to comply with his orders. The patient has a right to refuse, but she becomes intimidated. You end up being the heavy, trying to explain the two opposing approaches while trying to keep the patient's trust. It's tricky.

We get a lot of contradictory messages from the physicians I work with. A physician, who will not allow a nurse to give a popsicle to the laboring patient without his written order, will say to me, "When you have to deliver any of my babies and I can't get there, make sure you do an episiotomy." That's an operative procedure he's trusting me with; only nurse midwives are trained to do episiotomies. The messages I get are, "Yes, you can do the medical interventions because I said so, but don't do nursing things because I didn't say so."

A really fresh memory is the stillbirth I delivered a few weeks ago. The mother's physician had diagnosed the fetal death a few days before she went into labor, and he had alerted the obstetrical nurses. She was stopped at the emergency room. The E.R. staff called and said, "Come down, we're having an emergency delivery." When I arrived at the E.R. I immediately recognized June. This was her second stillbirth. I said, "Let's get her upstairs quick." The E.R. doctor said, "Not until I get heart tones." June knew her baby was dead. I pulled the doctor aside and told him that there had already been a confirmation of the fetal death. No heart sounds had been obtained by ultrasound for over a week. But the doctor continued to insist on placing a fetal monitor before he'd allow us to take June to the delivery room. We called the nursing manager, but she refused to take action.

So, we got a monitor on the patient. The doctor placed the Doppler [device used to test for fetal heart tones] around her abdomen, stopped, and said, "Is that the heartbeat?" Since he wasn't an OB, he didn't know anything about monitoring. What he was hearing was the mother's pulse. The couple, who had previously acknowledged the baby's death, started to have false hope. After several minutes of fishing for the heartbeat, he gave up. It was really cruel for him to get their hopes up just so he could show his stuff.

Shortly after we got the lady to the delivery room, I delivered a stillborn child. Later, her physician called to ascertain if she was in the hospital. I said, "You *know* she's here and the baby is here, too." I knew the emergency room staff had already called him. He'd had a particularly hard time with pregnancy loss. We all do. We go into this to bring life, not death.

The baby was beautiful. I baptized the baby as the mother had asked. The footprints were taken. Both parents held the lifeless baby.

The parents wanted the younger children to see and hold the baby. It wasn't something the chaplain or physician had encouraged. It wasn't something that I'd personally do, but since it was what they wanted, we went along with their wishes. The chaplain and physician left.

It was midmorning, and the children didn't come to see their sibling until suppertime. Though it was several hours past the time I was off duty, I stayed to see the family through. It wasn't fair to them or the staff for me to leave. The kids didn't know the baby was dead. They came bobbing in, expecting to see their newborn brother. The oldest child had written a note to the baby that morning, saying she'd be the best big sister ever. The younger child didn't want to hold the baby. He just looked. When the family seemed stable, I left them alone to grieve in privacy. They called me when they were done. I gave the younger child one of the baby's identification bracelets, and I gave the older one the cap and a lock of hair. She held the baby. I took a picture of her and the baby for her bulletin board. The image I still hold is of this gorgeous little girl, smiling down at her dead baby brother.

The younger child was so frustrated that he slammed his hand into the mattress. I suggested that he needed a hug. The dad quickly took him into his arms. Those kinds of instances are definitely nursing. I hope we never lose it.

Nurses are fighting for their right to do nursing care. The movement is slow. The labor room is not the place to confront the physician with what one's role is or is not. We pull back. Otherwise, the physician may retaliate on the patient. Just the other day, a patient refused an enema, and the physician got mad and delayed starting the pitocin to induce labor. He was angry because the patient had defied his orders, so he decided she'd have to wait. If I had confronted the physician with his defiant behavior at that crucial time, the patient would have received the brunt of his anger.

In institutions where there is shared governance, both physicians and nurses get together periodically to clarify their roles and develop procedures. The institution I work in doesn't have shared governance. The physician has a lot of power and the hospital is giving the "high-admitter" doctors even more say, just to keep them there.

In this type of setting, the nurse learns to manipulate. If we know that the doctor will only give pain medication to patients whose cervix is dilated five centimeters and above, we'll fudge. If the patient is four centimeters and contracting strongly, we'll tell the physician she's at five. Sure, you're stretching the story, but you've learned through experience that the medication will relax the patient and speed labor. After you've coached her to get through the hard part, sometimes she needs the medication to relax enough to let nature run its course.

I've seen hundreds of patients throughout their labors; the physician hasn't. He hasn't been with these women or had the opportunity to test the accelerating effect of medication on labor. He's gone through a very rigid training system, and he's lost if he doesn't follow a set sequence of steps.

Physicians often look at convenience. They have office practices and they'd prefer the patients to deliver to accommodate their schedules. They don't see the harm in delaying the birth process for a half hour or so. Then you've got the opposite, such as the doctor who intervenes with an epidural anesthetic at four centimeters so the patient will progress rapidly.

We nurses juggle a lot of personalities and preferences. The unit works differently depending on which nurse is on duty. Nurses who are openly assertive are labeled aggressive bitches. Once the physicians label you aggressive, no one wants to work with you. You've lost your credibility.

You can continue to be assertive and insist on doing the nursing things, but the physicians will challenge every decision you make. For instance, a woman can "push" in a variety of positions. She can push the fetus while she is standing, sitting, or lying down. If the physician believes she can only push lying down and he walks in when a woman is pushing in a standing position, he'll question the practice. Unless you have a quick answer, such as, "The baby wasn't coming down well, so we're going to try this position," the physician will demand she lie down.

Part of the attitude is due to the nurse managers who fail to support their staff nurses. When the physician confronts the nurse manager, shouting, "Can you believe what your nursing staff is doing!" the manager had better have a quick answer or she's as much as admitted that she's incapable of defending her nursing staff. By feeding into the physician's scenario, a manager can limit what nurses choose to do. The overlaps between nurses and physicians are not acknowledged.

I believe that these physicians try to control our practices because they are threatened. If we demand our practice rights, the patients will realize that most of what they need is nursing. That's certainly the case with the majority of obstetrical patients. The birthing centers have proven that. If the patient gets smart, she'll ask, "Why am I paying fifty dollars for an office visit, when I can have the same and more for less money from a nurse midwife?"

Another realistic fear of the physician is a malpractice suit. If roles aren't clear-cut and something adverse occurs due to the nurse's action, the physician may be held accountable. Social policy needs to be redefined to clearly give the nurse responsibility and authority for her actions.

I'm torn when I have to deliver the baby when no doctor is present. Legally, I run a lot of risks, yet I can't leave a helpless woman. I stick my neck out and do the delivery or the episiotomy. I do that knowing full well that somebody could sue me.

We have no resident staff. Even though we are a low-risk unit, the unexpected emergency occurs. The nurse has to handle it. A while back, I had a patient whose baby's fetal heart tones suddenly dropped way down to eighty. On pelvic exam, I could feel the cord in front of the baby's head. The cord had prolapsed. When that happens, you have to act fast. I called the woman's obstetrician, the operating room, and the anesthetist. By the time the obstetrician walked in, the team was ready for a cesarean section. That kind of split-second teamwork doesn't always occur fast enough. If the physician doubts the nurse and insists on coming in to diagnose the case himself before getting the operating room set up, precious time is lost.

One particular physician never listens to others. One time, he called me and said, "I'm sending a patient in with three-minute contractions. She says they're hard, but I don't think they are. The baby was breech the last time I saw her." I said, "Why don't you come in; it sounds like she's ready to deliver." He said, "No, you check her when she comes in and call me."

The emergency room nurse brought her up in a wheelchair, and I could hear her grunting before I even saw her. We quickly got her on the delivery table and checked her. At that point, the membranes ruptured and old meconium gushed out, signifying the fetus had been in dire distress. Next came the baby—blue, without a heartbeat. The E.R. nurse and I resuscitated the baby. After a few minutes, we got a heartbeat and placed the baby in the warmer.

When the nursing supervisor arrived, she could only criticize. She groused that the wheelchair didn't belong in the delivery room. Then she challenged my authority to give pitocin. The lady had been bleeding, and I'd taken the situation into my own hands.

When the physician came, he acted surprised and said, "What happened?" I thought, "*What* happened? *You* didn't come to the hospital when you knew a multipara was in labor!"

He had the nerve to say to the mother, "Yeah, the nurse says the cord was tied around the legs, but I've never seen that"—intimating I didn't know what I was talking about. At that point, I turned to him and sarcastically said, "You could have seen the first one if you'd been here." Later, the mother told me that she didn't know how the doctor could doubt me when it was obvious, from the looks of the baby's legs, that the cord had definitely been constricting them. Surprisingly, the baby did well mentally, although his lower legs are still disproportionate to the rest of his body.

We need to have a way to give more care by the same person to OB families. Sometimes, you work a whole shift with a family, and the laboring mother has gotten to trust you, and then your shift is over. We need to figure out a way to establish a fee for service in which the nurse follows the patient until completion.

A while back, I was told I had too altruistic an attitude, that I'd have to smarten up. The nursing supervisor told us, "The caring things are no longer able to be paid for." I can't stand to hear that. I'd leave nursing if that happened. What we have that's special is our caring. If we lose that, we have nothing.

6

In the Dead of Night

Mental health institutions are not equipped to care for patients who are physically ill. Sara works in a hospital unit that makes special provisions for mentally disturbed patients.

Imagine a mother figure and she would be Sara: soft, compassionate, warm. She meets us at eight A.M., *when her night shift is completed. Her uniform is no longer fresh, and there is a touch of fatigue about her eyes.*

Sara appreciates the independence of working nights; experienced nurses like it that way. The hall lights are dimmed, the pace shifts to low gear and, as Sara puts it, "If you have any intelligence at all, people let you do things without bothering you."

I've been an employee of County Hospital for twenty years. I started out when I was nineteen, washing glassware in the hematology lab. I'm the type who always wants to learn more. I went on and trained to be a lab technician. Most of the time, I've worked nights.

On the psych floor, there aren't any doctors around at night. For the most part, I'm on my own. I draw on a lot of my physical assessment skills and my lab knowledge.

On the night shift, patients are lonely. Their families aren't there—no one is. Even when the family can be there, the patient is the one who is sick and no one else. If a person has someone caring and friendly around, it makes a difference in how he or she feels.

Patients who come to my psychiatric floor have both mental problems and something physically wrong, such as broken bones, cancer, pregnancies, or med-surg problems. I function primarily as a psych nurse. I help them get in touch with their feelings; I talk with them so they understand the effects of what happened to them in the past. Many will come in with abdominal pains or lower back problems, and you'll find that rape, incest, or other types of physical abuse are the underlying problems.

For instance, one of the patients was raped when she was seventeen. She decided that she was ruined for life and she married the rapist. For years she put up with his sexual abuse. "He entered every orifice of my body," she told me. He did everything you could imagine—he did a number of abortions on her, strung her up in the barn and abused her with a cattle prod. The night she first told me about all this, we sat and talked a long time. She was in her fifties, and all this time she had kept it to herself. She hadn't told her family or anyone else back home.

Her husband had ruined her physically. She was repeatedly admitted to our floor with pelvic infections. The doctors figured she was abusing herself and couldn't figure out why she didn't stop. Because she had confided in me, I was able to explain her situation to the doctors.

Finally, her husband raped her sister. My patient wouldn't testify at his trial, but it did bring her to her senses. She got a divorce.

She was readmitted to our unit two months ago with a minor problem. She'd remarried—to a man with three children. She couldn't have children, and his children became like her own. Last summer, he began going out with other women. This triggered all the anger and hostility she'd kept inside for over thirty years. She told me that, at home, her new kitten soiled a floor she had just cleaned and, in a rage, she beat it to death. To do such a bizarre thing . . . she'd lost touch.

On our unit, her fury and anger were expressed in nightmares. I used imagery to relax her after she'd had them.

When I asked her to imagine a peaceful scene, she couldn't. Her image of something peaceful was a little girl in a white dress skipping in the woods where the leaves were burning. The scene reminded her of a time when she was badly burned as a small girl. Her sister happened to light a match while their mother was using kerosene to treat my patient for hair lice. Once she talked about her nightmare, she was able to share her problems with her new marriage. It helped her progress.

We had another patient who came in with all sorts of unexplained pains. She'd been sexually abused by her grandfather when she was four years old. Then her father started sexually abusing her. She had been in and out of the hospital many times before all this came out. She had an abusive uncle who followed her until she was seventeen. He used to tie her down. She sold drugs to a motorcycle gang as a way to invite gang rape. It was the only means she could see to get love.

She told us nurses of her experiences—blandly, without expression. She showed no anger. I said to her, "If someone did those things to me, if people hurt me like that, I would be angry. It's okay to be angry, you know." Soon—well, not really *soon*, in a little while—she started to get the anger out. She was finally able to express it.

When the doctors came around, she would be manipulative and flirtatious. She would be humped over in bed with pain. When female nurses were around, she behaved like a normal person without physical problems.

Doctors see the patient maybe fifteen minutes a day—or less—but we're there and see behavior over the twenty-four hours. The lady may convince the doctors she is physically sick, but nurses who are there all day can assure the doctor that she is just fine. The team can use that information to conclude that the patient is attempting to create overdependence on her psychiatrists.

Among nurses, passing information from shift to shift, day to day, is important. Patients will distort information to get attention. One shift will report, "The patient said he had a heart attack," and then the next shift nurse will say, "The patient says he had a coma." You realize what the patient is trying to do. On our psych floor, we consider behavioral symptoms much more significant than the physical.

Psychiatry doesn't give instant rewards. Changes in patients' behaviors are gradual. It usually takes months, if not years, to make a difference.

My most memorable patient was a drug-addicted, pregnant nurse. She said she started using drugs because she'd been raped. Her husband was driven crazy by the thought of that, and he couldn't stand the pregnancy, either. She complained of excruciating abdominal pain. No one would believe her; they couldn't find the cause of her pain. She supposedly had been off drugs since before the pregnancy, but they didn't trust her.

I decided that the pain couldn't be a put-on. There are definitely manipulative patients, but I knew this wasn't one because of what she was going through. We gave her all kinds of medication, but it didn't end the pain. Finally, all I could do was sit there and hold her. To me, that's what nurses are there for—the comfort, the human touch. The doctor was there, but all he would do is order medications. When you have patients who are dying or suffering terribly, what they want most is for someone to be there—to touch them and be with them.

7

Home Hospice Nurse

As shadows soften in the evening dusk, Linda's strong, clear voice carries us back, to a time five years ago when she was a hospice nurse. The vividness of her recollections causes tears to surface, yet they are fleeting. Her acceptance of grief keeps her serenity intact.

Being a hospice nurse represents the best two years of my nursing career. I could tell that what I did made a difference to the patients. Before that, I'd been working in pediatrics, rotating to nights every other week.

An opening came up in hospice to work days. I'd always liked the hospice idea. They were looking for a nurse who was comfortable making her own decisions. They asked me, "What would you do if you had a patient in pain? Suppose you couldn't contact the physician for a narcotic order? How would you manage?" I was impressed that they were interested in my problem-solving ability. To be honest, though, the real motivator in taking the job was getting off the night shift.

Oh, I can't say I wasn't leery of the job. After all, I was only twenty-two and fairly fresh out of school. I wasn't sure I could face the magnitude of those patients' needs at such a critical time in their lives. It was such a big responsibility. It felt like we were the only ones there who were truly speaking up for them.

The job was in one of the first hospice home care programs. We nurses didn't give patients routine physical care, but we coordinated it. Coordinating meant organizing everything that had to do with the patient's home care. If the family needed special equipment, such as a wheelchair or walker, we would get it. We assessed any of the symptoms relating to the disease and took action. If the patient had a bowel impaction or a sore that wouldn't heal, we found it and took care of it.

Since patients at home needed care twenty-four hours a day, we taught the family how to give it. Home health aides and other services were available to the family. Someone could be hired to go in and relieve them if they needed to get away for a while, but the brunt of the care was on the family.

All hospice patients were expected to live less than six months, and the majority died at home. Rarely did the patient go back to the hospital. If they did, it was to receive chemotherapy or radiation for symptom relief, not to cure the disease.

By the time the patient contacted us for hospice care, his needs were strictly nursing. He no longer could be cured. His primary care was no longer given by a physician.

People misinterpret the philosophy of hospice. Some have the mistaken idea that everyone has given up on the patient. That's not so. Our goal in the hospice was to help patients live their lives to the fullest. Practicing physicians see a wholly different world when they're exposed to the way hospice nurses care for patients at home. I was free to make my own professional decisions. That was one reason I liked working hospice. The physician's attitude was, "If you can keep this family off my back, you can do absolutely anything within the bounds of safety."

Many of our patients had not been able to live with any quality of life prior to entering the hospice care program. Once they were pain free, we could get them out of the house, out to dinner. We helped them do things they thought they'd never do again.

One of my patients—I'll call him Dan—had extensive cancer, along with cardiac problems. The cancer had spread to his bones, resulting in multiple fractures, which was quite painful. Until we took over, he hadn't been able to get out of the house for months.

Dan loved to go out to dinner. In fact, we went out the night he died. He needed the help of the family and myself. I made him my last case of the day, and we all pitched in to get him ready to go out. He had several draining wounds that had to be bandaged, and you had to be careful moving him, as he easily fractured.

We all sallied forth to Dan's favorite bar and restaurant. Dan traded wisecracks with several of his old cronies, had a few drinks, and went home. That night, he died. He was a neat guy who fought to live his life fully.

Jimmy was another fellow I used to go to lunch with a lot. Sounds like I was always going out to eat with my patients! I was, but then, going out for some people was a big deal. Patients were afraid to leave their homes without a medical escort. They felt safe if the nurse went along.

You weren't supposed to take patients in your car, so I'd drive Jimmy's. He'd been in bed a long time, and he just expected to retire to bed and die there. It was as if he needed somebody to tell him that it was okay to go out. Jimmy had been a successful businessman, and it perked up his ego to be able to take the nurses out.

I guess you think I want everybody to get out of the house. Actually, if they can, it's the best thing for them. Today, people with cancer can die in relative comfort. It isn't like the old days—the cancer wards you'd read about, where people were screaming with pain.

People don't always interpret things like going out to dinner as nursing things. People consider these as "good person acts," not nursing. It's a combination of both, actually. If I hadn't understood Jimmy's physiology and the limits of his endurance, we couldn't have taken him out to lunch or given him so much morphine. Those decisions take nursing knowledge. In lots of patient situations, there were extra caring things that I'd do. Not every nurse is free to do those things. I know I can't put myself out that much now. However, at that point in my life, the hospice job was a twenty-four-hour-a-day commitment.

Nurses would share a call schedule. Patients knew they could call us anytime—day, night, and on weekends. They rarely called unless it was absolutely necessary. If a patient of yours died when you weren't on call, the call nurse phoned you anyway. I wasn't on call the night Dan died and the nurse neglected to call me. I was very upset, because I would have liked to have been there. I felt that Dan and I had unfinished business.

Occasionally, there were families that couldn't cope at all. They'd call at all times of the day and night. Or there was the occasional family that resented having to care for the patient. Maybe the patient's hospital insurance had run out, so the family was stuck with the care at home. They'd call the nurse for just about anything. On the whole, though, families coped surprisingly well.

I was constantly impressed by people's courage. A particularly brave Hispanic mom had a little girl with biliary atresia [a narrowing of a bile duct to the liver]. Baby Maria had a two-and-a-half-year-old brother and a father living in the home. The father, in his grief, separated himself from the child. He was unable to be supportive to the mother.

The child had a colostomy. The mother hauled this child back and forth every day for her hospital treatments. Maria was pathetic. You know how they get a yellow-green look from bile backup into their system? But this was this mother's baby, her little girl, and nothing was too much for her.

I spent most of my time preparing the mother for the signs of impending death, suggesting how she could handle the situation. Her child died at home in the ugliest way possible—she bled to death. Yet the mother was so happy to be there for the child at the end.

I'll never forget the day Maria died. It was very hard on me. I'd had three other patients die that day. I remember having dinner guests that night, and I sort of floated through the evening like a zombie.

Some patients in home hospice choose to go to the hospital to die. Once they are totally incapacitated, they don't want their families to be burdened any longer. That's okay, too. Sometimes, though, getting admitted to in-patient can be tricky. Medicare will only cover hospitalization of home hospice patients who demonstrate a medical need unrelated to the cancer.

For example, a person might have a cardiac condition that requires a pacemaker. Hospital personnel sometimes find this odd. They ask, "If the fellow is dying anyway, why treat his other medical problems?" They don't realize that people want to be up and around as much as possible. Cancer isn't always the only limiting factor; there can be other disease conditions as well.

I recall Joseph, a man who had a heart irregularity which was quite limiting. He admitted himself to the hospital to get his heart regulated. He also asked for a "no code" [no cardiopulmonary resuscitation], should he die. The physician and staff thought this was inconsistent, but it wasn't. Joseph was saying, "I know I have terminal cancer, and if I stop breathing, that's how I want to go. In the meantime, if you can straighten out my heart until the cancer gets me, then I want that done."

There was one lady who was admitted to the hospital because she had cervical cancer with metastases and a spinal-cord compression from the tumor. The lady was in excruciating pain. Jerry was a single woman who couldn't speak up for herself. She couldn't demand; she was too sick. She couldn't even get out of bed by herself. Her brothers came and forcibly took her to their home. They took away her autonomy—made her decisions for her.

The brothers insisted she have a catheter inserted. She didn't want that; she just wanted to die. She called me from her new residence, crying pitifully. In her own home she'd done what she wanted, whether others thought it was good or not. I personally didn't agree with the way she was taking care of herself, but that's the way she wanted it and I respected it. She lived on the ocean, and she enjoyed just sitting and looking at the waves. She'd sit on her couch, facing the ocean view, her medications and drinks on the table at her side. She was incontinent of urine. She had a pile of thick cotton pads in front of her. When she got wet, she'd haul herself up with tremendous effort, fling the wet pad out, and plop a dry one in.

At her brothers' home, she couldn't control anything;

she couldn't enjoy her ocean. It was really pathetic. She'd never married, and she prided herself on controlling her own life. At the end, she lost the control that was so precious to her.

Another pathetic elderly lady had a draining breast wound for years. She hid it from her daughter, who was a high society type with a husband who was an officer in the military. Pauline was ordinary middle class. When her daughter found out that she had this wound, the daughter insisted she get medical help. It was cancer—inoperable by this time. We nurses made home visits, packed Pauline's wound with sterile dressings. The next day, we'd find that she'd removed the dressings and applied her own home-style rag bandages. She claimed they were more comfortable.

She was on medications, which I'm sure she trashed. She didn't want anything done. It became a challenge to let her do things her way. We really conspired with Pauline against her daughter. Rather than fight the headstrong daughter, we let her think we were complying with her wishes. The day Pauline could no longer fight her daughter was the day she died. Against Pauline's will, the daughter admitted her to the hospital. Pauline died on the X-ray table.

I've learned a lot about letting people do things their own way. At first, I did what I thought was best for patients, regardless of their wishes. Nurses' personal value systems often get in the way of the patients' own wishes for their care.

For example, we hired a temporary relief nurse to come in and relieve a man who was caring for his wife. He hadn't been out of the house in several weeks. The relief nurse was extremely religious, and she believed in maintaining life at all costs. She didn't bother to check with the patient or husband about their wishes. She was, in fact, reading the Bible to the patient when the patient stopped breathing. The nurse started resuscitation procedures. She called the paramedics. They took the patient to the hospital, where they placed her on a respirator. It was simply bizarre. Here you had a terminally ill person, and they carted her off to place her on a respirator. We had a devil of a time convincing hospital personnel it was okay to take the lady off the respirator.

All of this occurred because the relief nurse's ethical values were imposed on a dying, suffering patient and her family. It was absolutely cruel. A regular hospice nurse would have let the lady die peacefully at home.

In hospice nursing, pain is a primary concern. We gave a lot of morphine and titrated the medication so the patient was continuously comfortable. Some hospital nurses have told me that they've used morphine for the patient and it doesn't work. If used correctly, in adequate amounts, it can work.

With the medicine available, there is rarely an excuse for uncontrollable pain. We'd titrate morphine in doses higher than normally recommended. Sometimes, a patient would get extremely sleepy, even comatose. You'd need to watch the vital signs very closely during that period, but it worked. It broke the pain cycle. The patient would think you were a miracle worker. Maybe, being so young, I was not afraid of risk. I wasn't afraid to administer that much morphine, but some nurses are.

It worked like magic. Patients stayed alert, left the house. I had one patient who drove his car, even after taking sixty milligrams of oral morphine. He wanted to get out and live during the time he had left.

Several patients received absolutely phenomenal amounts of morphine. One guy, Kevin, received two hundred milligrams every three hours at home—twenty times the normal dose. Then a horrible thing happened to him. He had to be hospitalized, and while he was there, he received only minimal doses of morphine. After five or six months of having received two hundred milligrams at a crack, five or ten milligrams just wasn't enough. He actually died of morphine withdrawal.

Even his physician, who had authorized the huge doses at home, refused to acknowledge Kevin's need for large doses in the hospital. I'm not quite sure why. Perhaps the physician was concerned his practice would more likely be questioned in a hospital, where other practitioners were around.

Unfortunately, a lot of hospitals still don't know how to handle pain as we do in hospice. A few months ago, I had a personal experience with my uncle, who died in the hospital. He had terminal liver cancer. A few days before he died, he became confused and combative. This is not unusual with the toxicity caused by the disease.

The hospital staff thought the confusion was a reaction to methadone, the drug he was getting, and they stopped giving it to him. The poor man just moaned and moaned. It took me, standing in the hall, shouting "Do something!" before they medicated him. They finally gave him Demerol and Vistaril, which hardly did anything for him. He continued to moan unbearably. I had gotten the physician to agree that my uncle could have a morphine drip started if his pain became uncontrollable. I asked the night nurse to start the drip. She refused, stating she didn't have the necessary supplies and she needed to contact the physician. Since it was one A.M., she refused to call him. I wanted to tell her to give me the equipment, that I'd do it myself, but I knew that from a legal standpoint she'd have to refuse. I wasn't on the staff and there would have been legal problems.

The doctor came at eight-thirty in the morning and the morphine drip was started about an hour later. My uncle had to bear his pain for over eight hours because of stupid hospital policies. I can't understand these things, nor can I forgive nurses who should speak up for patients and not just keep the rules. If my uncle had been at home, I could have relieved his pain immediately.

It required the constant presence of my aunt, my cousin, and me—all of us defending my uncle. The hospital nurses didn't like or appreciate any of us. They called my aunt "the witch" because she'd put up such a stink when my uncle was first admitted.

He'd had an I.V. going. Now, mind you, it had taken about fourteen sticks to get the needle placed at home. The hospital personnel wanted to restart it. The hospital policy said that all people admitted with I.V's should have them restarted. I guess it had to do with some legal issues. Anyway, my aunt actually stood in the doorway, keeping people from getting to my uncle to take out the I.V. She won, but they labeled her "the witch."

The nursing staff really let my uncle down; it was the doctor who was our knight in shining armor. We would convince him that certain things were needed for my uncle, and he'd order them.

Continuing to work with the dying was hard at times. I got a lot of support from my patients and their families. I remember talking to hospice volunteers once and having them ask, "How do you cope?" I said, "These people become my friends. When it is time for them to die, you've already worked through so much together. You're sure everything possible has been done. The patients and their families are comfortable that this is so. It's sort of an acceptance of the inevitable."

The fact that the person was dying was not the hard part. You were sad and cried a lot when they died, but it was tears touched with relief. The hard parts were the fights with hospital nurses, trying to get things for those patients. Those were the hurts. The hard part was not being able to change the world so these people could have what they needed to be comfortable.

8

Working with Cancer

It is twenty-five minutes past our interview appointment time. We wait at the nurses' station. Though it is long past the time the day-shift nursing staff should have been on their way home, several nurses are still finishing up.

Down the hall, a middle-aged patient shuffles along, pushing her intravenous equipment. Her blond hair is sparse, balding at the crown, mostly from the effects of cancer chemotherapy.

We ask if anyone has seen Bridget, and we're told she is giving change-of-shift reports and will be with us shortly. A few minutes later, she appears. In her mid-twenties, Bridget has sparkling eyes and is unmistakably Irish.

I really can't say I always wanted to be a nurse. I suppose, if I were to trace it back, I'd have to say that my interest in nursing stemmed from my experience with my brother, who had leukemia and died when I was in grade school. I remember the nurses being very kind to our family. The need to go into nursing must have been planted in my subconscious. In college, when the time came to declare my major, I gravitated into nursing. This is my first and only job since I graduated six years ago.

I wanted to work here at this hospital because I had my training here, and because it is a Catholic hospital. The philosophy here is consistent with mine. People in this hospital believe in a humanitarian approach to care. We have a well-run floor because the nurses, aides, and secretaries support each other. There are a lot of friendships among the staff, and a lot of patients want to come back to this floor because they feel this closeness. I guess you don't work on an oncology unit if you can't work with others. If you try, you don't stay there very long.

I didn't want to go into oncology nursing because of the experience with my brother, but it was the only opening in the hospital. At first, I tried to stay away from the leukemics and the younger people—especially the kids who were my brother's age when he died. I eventually discovered that the leukemics had very special needs, and I got involved in their care. There is always some new treatment, and a feeling of anticipation that a cure will be found. It is rewarding to work in that atmosphere—it brings an element of hope. Back in 1976, when my brother was sick, there was no hope for children with his type of leukemia. It is completely different now. Children sometimes have very long remissions, or even cures.

Cancer nursing is hard work, physically and mentally, but it isn't as bad as you'd think. You kind of get refueled because you feel you have done something for someone else. We get a lot more from situations than we put into them. It's not something you would want to miss. These patients make you feel that you're a good person.

Our supervisor thinks some of us get *too* involved. She thinks we go beyond the call of duty. I don't agree. When people are hurting, you can't just cut it off at the end of a shift.

My friend Judy and I became really close to several young men from Mexico. All three of these Mexican fellows were here illegally. They came to this country before there was such a big push to prohibit illegals. All had leukemia, and two of them have died. These fellows had very few family members here in the States, so they were kind of rootless and had no one else to look after them. If there hadn't been anyone to speak up for them, they'd have gotten lost in the system. So Judy and I took them under our wings, and we tried to help them as much as we could.

Jose, the last boy to die, was here without family support. He had a brother here, but the brother was sort of shiftless, drank a lot, and was not too dependable. Jose's last wish was to see his parents. Judy and I, along with a lot of other people in this hospital, were able to have the family with him for about a month and a half before he died.

It took a lot of work to arrange to get the money and visas for Jose's parents. Judy and I approached our head nurse about the problem. The director of nursing even enlisted the help of the hospital administration to contact the immigration services and use their influence. They got in touch with the Red Cross and a Hispanic agency that helps get emergency visas. Jose's doctor wrote a special letter pleading the case for the dying boy.

Jose was hospitalized for about eight months, and he touched the hearts of a lot of people. We have a lot of Mexican workers in our housekeeping, maintenance, and dietary departments, and they made a radio appeal over the Spanish-language station and raised about seven thousand dollars.

It's interesting how adversity brings out the best in people—suddenly, Jose's selfish brother became reliable. He took the initiative and went down to the border crossing in Texas, met the parents, and put them on the plane to Chicago.

We all got really close to Jose. It was very hard to watch him die. It was especially hard for me.

Watching people die is not easy, especially if the patients are close to your own age. We nurses talk about it among ourselves. Funny thing is, at first it seems so unfair when people die in their prime and will never be able to fulfill their dreams, but eventually you see death as an answer to their physical problems. Then it doesn't seem so unfair—it's just a release. It's harder to see them suffer than to see them die.

The ability of families to cope with the patients' situations varies widely. Some do beautifully and others are totally unprepared. Sometimes, a member of the family denies the illness, and then it's difficult for them to give adequate care to the patient at home. See, we're not a hospice. Mostly, the patients without complications from the cancer are just sent home after chemotherapy.

Chemotherapy drugs are very potent. We don't administer them directly; there is a special team for that. They wear gloves and masks to prepare the drugs, and preparation is done under a laminar air flow hood.

We nurses on the unit take special precautions in disposing of equipment that has been exposed to the drugs. Some studies show that workers who are exposed to the drugs have some of it in their urine. There is potential drug absorption from handling patient waste over time, and there is still so much to learn about the long-term effects of handling the drugs.

We're involved in patient care in a way that isn't true of most health workers. If people in another department have a patient problem they can't solve, they come to the nurse. We get everything together into an effective care plan for the patient.

It's not in our job description, but I find that we do a lot of checking up on other people. For instance, the doctors order blood to be drawn early in the day, and often they don't get back to the patient until late afternoon or evening. They're in the clinic or in surgery. We usually look over the blood values as they come back from the lab. I'll call the doctor and tell him if the hemoglobin is dangerously low, and then he'll order blood or what-have-you over the phone. This way, we can get the therapies started early. We don't keep patients up all night.

I think reporting abnormal blood values is a nurse's role. You wouldn't want to let something go that would harm the patient just because it wasn't in your job description.

We try to accommodate families. If a patient is dying, we usually place the patient in a private room. We don't restrict visitors. Anyone who wants to be there, stays. Sometimes, there are as many as ten or twenty people present at the death. Not all of them can get into the patient's room at one time, so they stay in the waiting room nearby and take turns.

A lot of good people work here. They carry out their

philosophies. For example, when Jose died, he had a bill of over a quarter of a million dollars, and the hospital absorbed much of that cost. Other places would have sent him to a county hospital.

A lot of nurses go out of their way to do their jobs, but so do a lot of social workers and people in administration—like in the case of the young Mexicans. Their bills were way overdue and some places would have shipped them out. Our business office sort of ignored the bills. It wasn't dishonest; they just didn't send the bills to a collection agency. The institution absorbed the cost. They can't do that for everyone, but they do it for some. You'd never know about it if you didn't work here.

PART TWO

MATTERS OF CONSCIENCE

All professions have a code of ethics that reflects societal values. People enter a profession with personal value systems that have already been shaped by their religious experiences and cultural backgrounds. Dilemmas occur when personal values clash with those of the profession and society.

For some nurses, life should be maintained at all costs. For others, the patient and family's wishes are the yardstick used in decision making. Some nurses act as observers in the system, neither asking for nor having a say in ethical decisions affecting patient care. Others champion patients' rights. A few take situations into their own hands.

Moral and ethical concerns play a major role in nursing, where critical decisions are made every day. Few decisions, however, are as dramatic as the one made by Dan, who opted to execute his personal values and pull the respirator plug of an elderly person rather than watch the man die a slow and perhaps inhumane death. For Dan, the moral dilemma had strong legal implications, and he is still paying for his actions today.

In Shelley's case, quality of life was also an issue, though she was on the other end of the argument. Shelley supported the preservation of life at all costs, and she reaped the scorn of her co-workers when her philosophy worked against the tacit agreement to resist using extraordinary measures to save a baby girl with a poor prognosis.

Many nurses face moral dilemmas on a daily basis. Joan, a nurse and administrator with Planned Parenthood, is a Catholic who also has to consider the teachings of her church; she ultimately accepts the strong philosophical belief of family planners that all pregnant women have a right to know that abortion is a choice.

The AIDS crisis, more than any medical crisis in the century, has forced nurses to come to grips with their own beliefs and fears. Nurses not only fear for their health in caring for patients affected with a disease about which much is still to be learned, but their personal beliefs about homosexuality and drug addiction complicate the issue and clash with their moral duty to minister to AIDS patients. Many nurses flatly refuse to work with AIDS patients, while others put aside their fears and beliefs in what can truly be described as "the spirit of heroism." In telling her story, Emily further defines the fine lines in this dilemma.

For nurses, matters of conscience, like illnesses themselves, come and go. It is the way in which they contend with moral and ethical concerns that further determines the humanity of the profession.

9

Dan

What first strike you are Dan's boyish good looks. He tells his story in a calm, controlled voice.

I went into nursing after a stint in the service. I can't say I always wanted to be a nurse. In fact, I didn't think about nursing as a career for me until my sister, a nurse, told me about the opportunities in nursing.

As a Catholic, I decided to pursue my education at a Catholic college. In school, I enjoyed my intensive care experiences, so I went into intensive care after graduation, and I've been there ever since. That's where I was when the situation occurred that cost me my license.

I was working in a cardiac intensive care unit. The patients who were brought in had suffered heart attacks, strokes, and the like. Often, they were essentially dead and brought back to life. It wasn't unusual for a person who had been in our unit for weeks to die. Dying like that, without dignity, seemed so unfair and inhumane to me. The families were put through all that emotional turmoil and expense—and for what? To be left with high bills and no loved one.

I'll admit I was getting burned out. I had asked for a transfer to the emergency room, but it hadn't come through yet. My biggest frustration was having no power in the system. I was supposed to take care of patients, deal with their families, be hopeful and supportive, and half the time I didn't even know what the plans for patients were. If you'd ask a doctor, he'd treat you like you were trying to butt in. He'd make you feel like you should stay in your place. I'm not trying to indict the doctors, but it gets pretty hard when patients and families ask questions such as, "What are your plans for me?" or "What do you believe my outcome is?" or "What is our family member's outcome?" and the doctor's response is "Do you trust me? If so, I'll do the worrying." What can the patients and their families say? They can't say, "No, I don't trust you." So, what they'd do is pump the nurses for information. I guess, to be honest, I was angry and frustrated for being put in that situation.

I recognize that the doctor goes into medicine to cure, not to have people die. If doctors can't deal with that fact, then someone else should handle the situation.

That's the situation we were in with this patient, Mr. Marx. He was seventy-eight years old and had suffered a severe stroke at home. The paramedics had resuscitated him and brought him to our hospital. He was placed on a respirator and given drugs to maintain his heart rate and blood pressure. He was well into his second week, and since he had not regained consciousness, a brain wave test was done to see what brain activity existed. He had some brain wave activity at that time.

His family—his wife and three daughters—visited daily. By the third week, they were getting worn down. They felt they weren't getting any answers. They wanted everything possible to be done for the patient, yet they also knew that he never wanted to exist like a vegetable, so they asked for a conference with the doctors to discuss what should be done. Should Mr. Marx's life-support system be withdrawn?

It was interesting to me that the conference was held without any of the nurses who were intimately involved in Mr. Marx's care present. None of us even knew about the conference. The nurse who attended had taken care of him only a few times.

When I began my shift that afternoon, I was told the committee had discussed Mr. Marx's case, and its conclusion was that hospital policy didn't allow removal of the life-support system. Actually, that wasn't so. It really was the physician's interpretation, rather than what the policy actually said.

I went into the room where Mr. Marx lay, and I stood at his bedside. His youngest daughter was standing at the other side of the bed. She was obviously distraught, with tears rolling down her cheeks. She was slowly stroking his arm, shaking her head. She looked me straight in the eye and said, "If I could, I would end this thing."

It hit me like a ton of bricks—though she didn't ask me to do anything—it was just that all the suffering came together and I put myself in her place. How would *I* have reacted to being at the mercy of others? You know, people who come here trust us to help them. Sometimes we can't. Sometimes, with our modern-day methods, we make things worse and structure situations that leave us with no way out. If Mr. Marx hadn't been resuscitated and placed on our life-support system, he would have died naturally, when the stroke happened.

Oh, sure, the family was initially hoping a miracle would occur, that he would walk out of the hospital. Now they were stuck in a situation that nobody could—or would—end. It was so unfair—undignified for the patient, unfair for the family.

I don't know why, but suddenly I knew what I was going to do. For a few minutes, I thought of the consequences for me, legally and professionally, but the thoughts just passed. Looking back, I can say that maybe I should have made my position known, or maybe I should have tried to get people to change their minds. This patient would have died eventually. I still don't know why I decided to hasten his dying at that time.

It was late afternoon, after the visitors had left. I went into the room and stood for some time at the bedside, just looking down at the patient. No one else was in the room. The only sound was the rhythmic whooshing of the respirator. I touched his arm. There was no movement. I watched the air being pushed from the respirator though his breathing tube. His chest rose and fell, rose and fell, in a slow, regular movement.

The other nurse was outside at the nurses' station where the monitors were located. I disconnected the alarm on the monitor. I remember disconnecting the breathing tube with one hand and stroking his arm with the other. In nursing school, we were taught that hearing goes last. If he could hear, I wanted him to know what I was doing and why. I talked to him. I told him, "I am disconnecting the breathing tube. You will feel no pain. Soon your suffering will be over." I watched to see if there was any sign that he heard me or knew what I was saying. There was none.

Even though the monitor alarm was disconnected, the nurse at the station could see a printout of his heart rate on the computer screen. She saw his heart rate sharply falling and rushed into the room. She yanked back the curtain and stopped in her tracks, taking in the scene. At first, she looked puzzled, as if she couldn't believe what she was seeing. Then, as if to clarify her perceptions, she curtly asked, "What are you doing?" I answered, "What do you think I'm doing?" She said, "I can't believe what I'm seeing." Then she left. But that's not how she told the story later on. . . .

Mr. Marx's heart rate diminished and stopped. I then called the resident, to have him pronounce the patient dead. I notified the family. They only asked if the patient had died comfortably. I could honestly answer, "Yes." I removed all the equipment and positioned him so he looked peaceful.

At the end of the shift, I saw the other nurse at the time clock. She looked at me and said, "I never want to see anything like that again." I assured her she never would.

That occurred in September. One night, the following January, I came in for a few hours to teach some patient classes. The same nurse approached me and said she and another staff nurse from our unit wanted to discuss some things with me. She invited me to join them for drinks. I had other pressing matters and declined the invitation. She persisted and I refused again. Later that evening, I got a call at home from the nurse, who said it was urgent that they see me. I then agreed to meet them at a local bar.

The conversation evolved to problems with patients and ethical concerns. The nurse who had witnessed my actions asked me why I was so upset about another patient who had recently died, when I had done what I had done to Mr. Marx. The other staff nurse played dumb and asked me just what was it I had done. Looking back, I think this was a setup. I stupidly told them exactly what I had done. The other nurse's husband, it turned out, was a detective on the police force. Who knows? He may have convinced her to take some action.

When we left the bar, they drove the same way as I did, even though they lived in the opposite direction. They must have gone back to the hospital and written me up.

A few days later, detectives came to the hospital and arrested me for first-degree murder. My attorneys plea-bargained, and the offense was reduced to a misdemeanor. I was accused of practicing medicine without a license. I didn't have the family testify, and I was prohibited from contacting them. Anyway, I figured they'd suffered enough already. I had to go before the Board of Nursing, which ended up revoking my license for one year. The Board stipulated that I must take a course in nursing ethics before I could reapply for a license, and I'll do that—I clearly understand the ethics involved. I'll be eligible to apply for a license next year.

Meanwhile, in reality, even with my license reinstated, I don't know if I'll ever be able to practice nursing again. Who would hire me?

I am currently enrolled in a master's degree program in health care administration. I hope to direct a health care facility in the future. I hope to have an impact on ethics policies in the future and make a difference that I was unable to make as a nurse. The ethical decisions will become more complex as our society grows and technology increases. We somehow need to make decisions that allow people to die with dignity and let their families go on without being devastated by the experience.

I don't regret what I did. Maybe it could have been

handled differently, but I don't believe that what I did was wrong. What I did was professionally inappropriate, but it was ethically and morally right. It was a compassionate act. I will believe that until the day I die. When I stand before God, I know He won't say, "You're a killer and should go to hell."

10

Silent Agreement

Some matters of conscience are related, in confidence, when one nurse trusts another. Shelley's predicament had occurred the week before we talked to her, and it had been festering inside her since then. She asked us to meet her in the hospital cafeteria. Over coffee, she revealed the source of her frustration.

I work in the Intensive Care Unit. When things lighten up in the ICU, we sub on the general pediatric floor. That's how it was that Sunday morning. There were no patients in the ICU, so I went out to help with the kids. I was working North, across from baby Krista's room.

Krista is a nine-month-old with a degenerative neurological disease who has been here since shortly after birth. No one seems to know what caused her problem. A few weeks ago, we were able to take her out of her room in a special chair with the respirator connected.

Anyway, I wasn't assigned to her, but I was working on the north corridor. She has had a lot of problems with periods of apnea [breath cessation] lately. Her respirator is hooked up to a red flashing light in the corridor, and when she stops breathing a flashing light signals. It also flashes at the nurses' station.

I saw the red light flashing and I went running into her room. She was turning blue. I called a code to summon the cardiopulmonary resuscitation team. Meanwhile, I started CPR. The team came immediately and we were able to bring her back.

After the commotion settled down, I could tell that the floor staff nurses were upset. Finally, one of them came up to me and said, "Well, you really did it now. Why didn't you let her go? Don't you know when to walk slowly to the phone?"

I felt bad, as though I had killed her—or worse. You know, legally you must call a code on a child who has brain activity. Krista wasn't brain dead at the time, but now it looks as if she's brain-damaged. She just stares into space.

Apparently, the nurses and house staff had a silent agreement to not to use extraordinary measures on the child. This whole place, from the heating engineers to the people in the business office, know this child. They've almost made her a pet. Sara, who works in medical records, brought her a beautiful ruffled dress last month. The maintenance guy makes his daily rounds to see how "his little girl" is coming along. I guess the floor nurses couldn't stand to see her deteriorate. I can see how they feel, but nobody told me of the unspoken plan, so I called the code.

Even if I had known of the staff 's desires, I don't know if I could have gone along with the idea. After all, who are we to take the law and God's will into our own hands? I believe that when God wants this child, He'll take her. We don't need to help her along.

Frankly, it isn't easy. I have been ostracized by everyone and I've been treated badly, as if I caused Krista's brain damage through neglect. I hate to think of going out on that floor again.

These are the things that wear me down—all this trying to second-guess other people. I came into nursing to help people, not to take all this crap, and from my own kind, too.

POSTSCRIPT: Krista died two weeks after our conversation.

11

Family Planner

Joan plunks down her bulging black leather purse and eases herself into the booth at the Town Eatery. As one of the regulars at this neighborhood oasis, she waves aside the breakfast menu and orders. Leaning back expansively, she asks, "Well, what do you want to know?" Without hesitation, she shares her perspective with us.

I've done a lot of things in nursing—oodles and oodles. Right now, I'm an OB-GYN nurse practitioner and administrator with Planned Parenthood. I've been there since 1973. I've stayed because I'm committed to women's health care. Planned Parenthood started out offering women's health care, and it's since broadened to include reproductive health care for men and women.

I'm also committed to consumers having some say in their health care, and Planned Parenthood allows us to foster that. I give the people I see enough information to make wise health decisions. They're usually decisions as to whether they want to achieve a pregnancy or not—and when.

Of course, I do physical assessments and prescribe methods of birth control. With the current epidemic of sexually transmitted diseases, I do a lot of screening and treatment for that. I see the physical examination, diagnosis, and treatment functions as being an adjunct—I do them because we have to. Our heavy emphasis is really on health education, increasing awareness, and raising issues—all those things.

We give much more information to patients than they would customarily get in a doctor's office. We allow the women to make choices. Some physicians will do a fairly detailed patient history; they'll sit down and ask maybe eight or ten pertinent questions and then do the pelvic examination. They'll write the prescription and send the patient to the drugstore without ever offering her a choice of contraceptive method. They may know that the patient smokes a pack-and-a-half of cigarettes a day, and suggest that she quit smoking, but I think "You ought to quit" is a lot different from "You need to consider how much you are smoking in relation to your birth control pills, because this is an additional risk."

Very often, women will come in and say, "The doctor gave me the prescription but he didn't tell me how to start the pills." That concerns me. You see women coming in on these extremely high dosage pills when they've never been on anything else. They'll get angry when you say, "You know, we really ought to be concerned about this high a dosage. Lower-dose pills are just as effective and are potentially much safer." They'll say, "My doctor put me on this."

"Well," I'll tell them, "I'm sorry your doctor put you on these, but my job is to give you health information. I don't know why you are on one hundred micrograms of estrogen. It's not going to change the effectiveness of preventing pregnancy. It's safer for you from the standpoint of heart attack, stroke, or blood clots if you were to start dropping your dose slowly every three months until we get to thirty-five micrograms. If you don't want to do that, fine. However, I'm noting on your chart that I have discussed this with you. I can't force you to do it."

All this reinforces the idea that this is serious business; it also covers my hind end. It says, too, if a chart is ever reviewed, that I am practicing wisely and giving the best care I can.

It's like when people come in for a pelvic exam. I look at the cervix and see all kinds of pus discharge. With chlamydia infections, it's one of the symptoms. The patient will say, "I don't need any screening for sexually transmitted diseases," and I'll tell her, "I would be giving you lousy care if I didn't screen you." She might give me a lot of heat about money, so I'll say, "Well, then, I won't charge you. I'm more concerned about giving you good care than collecting money."

An older woman came in one time who had questions about menopause. She told me that she had come back because I'd taught her how to do a breast exam. She'd been checking and had found a lump. She had come back because I'd given her information about her body that she never received anywhere else.

When a woman who is trying to conceive comes in, we find out how much she knows about her fertility pattern. If she doesn't know a lot, we start her out with some easy reading; then we plug her into some fertility method and our family planning classes. If she's been trying to achieve a pregnancy for a year, and if it seems as if she's been doing her timing well and still can't conceive, I'll refer her to an infertility specialist. I'll give her a little rundown on what to expect from a fertility physician before she goes.

Some physicians have a problem with us prescribing contraceptive drugs. That's the old issue of others "diagnosing and treating" what physicians think is their domain. The state allows it under a stringent set of protocols. The protocols are signed by a statewide medical director, and they cover all of our clinic sites.

I just can't get caught up in physicians' problems with nurses prescribing drugs. Nurses have been making decisions on which drugs to use since the early sixties.

In 1966, I worked in an intensive care unit where we were shooting lidocaine into I.V.'s to regulate patients' hearts. We had no standing orders, no protocols—no nothing. The physicians didn't want to staff the ICUs around the clock, so they told us to go ahead and decide when and how much to give.

So I guess I've always been on the cutting edge. I've also refused to follow a physician's orders a time or two. I was never one to say, "Well, I'll do it because he has these magical initials after his name."

For instance, I refused to pull an IUD on a pregnant patient in an outlying clinic last month because one of the risks was that she might have aborted right there. My medical director told me that I should, and I said, "Nope, I'm not comfortable with it," at which point he said, "Fine, then send her in to me at the main clinic."

I've asked myself if I could work for Planned Parenthood if I wasn't committed to its philosophy. I don't think so. I think I would be miserable, and I think the people around me would be miserable. I cry with my patients and I rejoice with them. One of the most difficult things I ever did in nursing was to take a dead baby out to the mom. I will never forget that . . . ever! It was very difficult.

I'd say that probably the most difficult situation we have to deal with is a teenager coming in, thinking she is pregnant, and finding out that she is. It seems that they're getting younger and younger. You see a scared fourteen-year-old standing there in her school T-shirt and loafers, and you have to tell her she's pregnant.

First, you have to get them over the crisis. You have to let them vent their feelings, whether it's just sitting and crying, hysterics, or swearing. Very often, the teen will say, "I didn't think this could happen." You wouldn't believe the misinformation they get—"It won't happen the first time you have intercourse," or "If you do it at such-and-such time of the month, you can't get pregnant." Very often, they have to deal with a lot of guilt. "If only I hadn't . . ."

Very often, too, kids don't want to tell their parents. Just think about the message all parents give. I don't know of any parent who tells his or her kid to go out and have sex. Parents say, "Don't do that." The message, whether they know it or not, is, "You'd better not come home and tell us you're pregnant."

Most kids come in without their parents knowing that they've come to Planned Parenthood. I always encourage them to tell their parents. I warn them that there will probably be a big row, but in the majority of instances, the parents are supportive and will continue to be. It's part of parenting. They may not agree with the decision about whether to continue the pregnancy, but that decision is ultimately the mother's, and it's always a difficult one.

Here are these kids, who have been involved in adult activities and are now faced with raising children—one of the most difficult adult activities there is. They have to make an adult decision when they haven't matured to that level. Yet, they are the ones who will always live with the consequences of their decision.

You get them to the point of at least realizing that they don't have to decide on the spur of the moment. I'll tell them, "You have to decide whether you're going to continue this pregnancy or whether you're going to terminate it. If you are going to continue the pregnancy, you'll have to do all the things that will bring a healthy outcome for you and the baby. That means early prenatal care, looking at habits that may affect the fetus. If you decide to have the baby, you'll need to decide whether you're going to raise the child or put the child up for adoption. You need to know what that involves. If you bring a baby into your life, how many of the fun things in school are you going to be able to do? Are you going to be able to concentrate on your assignments after you've been up all night because the baby's sick or teething or doing those other things that babies do? On the other side, if you decide you're going to terminate the pregnancy, you'll need to look at where you should have your abortion procedure and progress from there. Who's your significant support person? Is your partner going to be involved in the decision-making process? Maybe a good friend—someone who's been in the same situation—could at least listen to you vent your feelings. You need to look at your life's goals, where you see yourself going. Are you going to be able to get through this by yourself?"

Of course, if the teen walks in and is already twenty-six-weeks pregnant, there is no choice at all. She must complete the pregnancy. You get into the question of why she waited so long to come in. She's missed her periods, she's feeling life inside her, and her physical shape has changed.

How can she *not* realize that this has been going on? She has no *choice* but to go home and tell her parents that she is pregnant and going to deliver shortly.

Not everyone can deal with teens who aren't telling their parents, just like not every nurse can deal with working in critical care or a hospice unit. We are people, like everyone else. We have biases, different family backgrounds, different religions. There are so many other options. Goodness sakes, why be miserable? I don't know why anybody would want to work in a situation they don't believe in. That's part of professionalism. I would hope that nurses would get themselves out before they could hurt someone.

I have two daughters—one who will be seventeen in January, and one who will be sixteen in February. They've grown up with Planned Parenthood materials, with me bringing home audio-visuals. They've seen graphic illustrations projected on the dining room walls when I've been preparing presentations for some group workshops.

In some instances, it's been difficult for them because we are Catholic. My kids are in a private Catholic high school, so they've learned to sift information. They know they can't wear their Planned Parenthood T-shirts to the church festival. I don't think that's bad. You have to learn to sift other kinds of information, and this is just another piece of that learning process. The neighborhood kids come to my daughters to ask questions because they know where I work. If the kids know you're okay, they'll seek you out—the guys as well as the young women. Our daughters have learned that not all their friends' parents think as we do. That's not good or bad; that's just the way it is.

Men are another one of my special interest groups. I like men, but I think they should be taking more responsibility when it comes to reproductive health. Society hasn't done much to give them that message. You'll see only a small number who will come in with their partners. These men want information, and they want to be involved in the decisions; they don't want their partners hurt or put in jeopardy.

Some men hesitate to come in, even though their partners are receiving treatment for sexually transmitted diseases. The men may not have the symptoms, and they can't understand why they have to take medicine if they don't have symptoms.

Some men come in just to buy condoms. Their friends have told them that we're okay, and sometimes it's cheaper. They may get their condoms for nothing because the price is figured according to poverty guidelines. On their first visit, they're usually a little nervous and shy. The second time, they're okay because they know we aren't going to hassle them. In some of the smaller clinics, you see a group of men on a regular basis. Very often, the staff can call them all by their first names.

Men are coming in more and more for screening for sexually transmitted diseases. They'll have a rash, a sore, a discharge, something they know isn't right. Once they get in and find out that ours is a safe environment, they're willing to ask questions that they've not been willing to even ask their friends.

Or a kid will come in for screening for sexually transmitted diseases and you'll see that he has a lifestyle in which he may not have known his partners very well. Now he's concerned. You give him some information about how to protect himself by using condoms. The next time you see him, he tells you he's using a condom, or that he's in a stable relationship. It's satisfying to know he won't end up getting a venereal disease.

The fact that our female practitioners examine men's genitalia doesn't seem to be much of an issue to the men. They're usually so concerned that they just want their problems fixed. They want to be treated with dignity and respect and get their questions answered.

Other nurses have asked me if I am pro-life. I don't know anybody who's *not* pro-life. I'm very much pro-life, but I want that life to be a wanted one. I want the decision that goes into it to be a responsible one.

I don't know what I would do if I was in the situation of an unwanted pregnancy, because I have never been there.

I do know that if I were there, or if my two teenage daughters were there, I would want them to have all their options explained to them.

I want women to have abortion as an option. I don't want that option taken away. Every woman who comes in for a pregnancy test is asked what she might do if the test shows that she is pregnant. I may say, "I see you've made the comment here that you intend to continue the pregnancy. What made you decide that?"

They may answer, "Well, I'm against abortion." I'll ask them what they mean by that, and they'll say, "It's killing a baby." I'll tell them that they need to be aware that abortion is a choice, and if they don't want to look at it as a choice, there are other choices to consider.

I guess I'm not sure if there is anything I'm going to say to them that would dissuade them if they firmly believe that abortion is killing a baby, that it's a life from the time of the fertilization of the egg in a woman's body. I can't say if it would abort along the way because there is an abnormality, but at least I've said, "You need to think about it; it is a choice for you."

There are situations where people will come in and say that they're going to continue the pregnancy. Then you'll see them two or three weeks later and they have had an abortion and are now looking for a method of contraception. I'll say something like, "I see you looked at your choices and made a decision different from the one you made here." Very often, they'll answer, "Yeah, I thought about it and realized I couldn't raise the child," or "I couldn't tell my parents, I couldn't destroy the trust my parents have in me." For those teenagers, living with the abortion decision is better, which is kind of too bad.

We worry about safety issues when packages arrive. Some Planned Parenthood clinics have been bombed. There has been picketing at some clinics. A couple of clinics in this city have had red paint thrown on their doors. These are nuisances but it has not been disruptive to service delivery stuff. Someday, we could have a pro-life sit-in, I suppose. We'll deal with it when it comes.

12

The Spirit of Heroism

Emily cares, without question, for patients with AIDS.

The unit I work on is a general medicine unit, in transition. Our patients include cardiacs, drug overdoses, alcoholics in DTs, and we take care of all AIDS patients in the hospital. If a patient with AIDS is admitted to another unit, the personnel grab the phone to see when a transfer can be made.

Yes, it's true—not everyone wants to nurse patients with AIDS. Even though a nurse is assigned to a person with AIDS, she can be cruel or refuse to go into the patient's room. There are some on our unit who absolutely refuse to care for AIDS patients. There are different reasons for their doing this. An overwhelming concern, obviously, is the fear of acquiring a disease that has no cure and is fatal. Others have religious objections. I work with a nurse who is very religious. She provides excellent care for the patients, but she refuses to care for AIDS patients because she feels they are sinners and deserve to die. I've had doctors refuse to start an I.V. on a patient with AIDS for fear of blood contamination. They are no different from the famous heart surgeon who said he wouldn't operate on an AIDS patient. In a way, it's legitimate. You need to be careful.

Recently, a news service reported that two hospital workers had become AIDS positive, seemingly through contamination from caring for AIDS patients. I reviewed that study carefully. Both of the people who were infected had skin diseases with open lesions. I believe it was preventable. If you work with blood products without wearing gloves, you can expect to be contaminated.

It was unfortunate that the story was leaked to the press. It was a blatant misuse of information. The day the story broke, someone placed the newspaper article on the bulletin board in the nurses' station. Immediately, we had nurses refusing to care for the AIDS patients. These nurses were very vocal in their negative commentaries. The article gave them false information to substantiate their biases.

Caring for AIDS patients is really no different from caring for anyone with a communicable disease. Unfortunately, over the years hospital personnel have become lax when caring for patients with communicable and contagious diseases. If you get a staph infection from a draining wound, you can always take an antibiotic; with AIDS, there is no cure.

The fact that many of the patients are homosexuals makes it difficult for some people to work with them. I personally find the person who acquired AIDS through drug abuse more difficult. On the whole, the drug abuser is more noncompliant with the treatment regimen. They'll lie or do a lot of other things to sabotage their treatment. It's frustrating, and I resent them. They take up a lot of time and space for something they inflicted on themselves. They'll probably hurt other people in the process of getting their own selfish needs met. I know they might all have mental problems, but I must admit I cannot be tolerant of these people. I see homosexual men differently, even though I don't understand their lifestyle.

I don't necessarily approve or understand any of the behavior that leads people to acquire AIDS, but that's not for me to judge. AIDS is different from other cancers. People suffer terribly and we should provide help.

I took care of the first patient diagnosed with AIDS in the state. Gerry practically bled out [slow hemorrhage] from his draining wounds. His whole immune system was shot. He developed overwhelming systemic infections, and the drugs used to treat them added to his problems. His blood wouldn't clot. He had diarrhea, and he had terrible sores in his mouth.

One of my most memorable patients was a drug addict. Her name was Sally. She'd apparently been a lady of the night, possibly to support her drug habit. Kaposi's sarcoma was on her heels and ankles, and the weeping lesions caused pain to the point where just placing sheets over her caused spasms of pain. Sally had pneumocystis [a type of pneumonia]—her lungs were filling up with fluid. Many of the respiratory therapists refused to provide her treatments. I didn't care, so I did the treatments. I couldn't see how you could watch someone drowning in her own secretions and not help her.

I cared for Sally the night prior to the morning she died. She was gasping for air. She was scared. Knowing she was dying, she pleaded with me not to leave her alone. When I had to attend to the other patients, I asked the L.P.N. [Licensed Practical Nurse] to sit with her. We changed her when she was incontinent, suctioned her, gave her pain medication, and soothed her.

I couldn't stop her death, but I made her as comfortable as possible. She asked me to pray with her. "I've never ridden the white horse before," she said, which is a saying from *Revelations.* "I need to pray, I need to make my peace. Can you help me pray?" She died the next morning. Just talking about it makes me feel sort of weepy and sad, but I'm glad I was there.

One of my favorite patients died at home. Chris was a honey. He had a support group to end all support groups. I mean, he had a huge collection of friends. He was very popular, a fun person. Chris talked a lot about his feelings to me. I was working nights, and I find that people tend to talk more personally at night.

"I don't know if I can get Dan"—his significant other—"to realize that I need to go now," he told me. "It's been too much for me." He looked sorrowfully at me and said, "Emily, do you think you can talk to him, make him realize I can't go on any longer?"

My tears started flowing. I told him I'd see what I could do.

I didn't know how I was going to approach the subject with Dan, but it just happened. Chris was dozing rather fitfully one afternoon, and Dan and I were sitting in the corner of the room, talking quietly. Dan asked me, "Emily, do you think it's getting to be the time?"

I said, "Yes, I think so. I think you need to let Chris know you are willing to let him go." Both of us started to bawl.

Chris opened his eyes and said, "Will you two stop your bawling? Would you mind not slopping over me?" His words broke the tension, and we wound up laughing and crying at the same time. Chris died at home a week later, with Dan at his side.

Relatives of AIDS patients react no differently from other relatives of ill people; some are supportive and some are not. We had one family that literally dropped the patient off. They said he was too much work for them to handle. He never saw his family again.

Some families are supersupportive. Sure, it's a shock to families. It's devastating for families to find out that their son had a lifestyle foreign to their own, and now he is dying, too. I recall a mother who found it very difficult to accept her son's homosexuality. She made sure I knew she'd raised a "straight" child. Yet she was extremely loving to the sick son. I think it's very difficult to disown your child. You may not approve of his behavior, but it's pretty hard to abandon him in his time of need.

You also have to realize that, just because people have AIDS and are dying, they are not martyrs or saints, nor are they being punished for their disease. Hell, it's a disease that doesn't have a cure, just as cancer doesn't have a cure. Both kill. AIDS moves a little faster.

People ask me why I'm involved with AIDS patients when I have a husband and a child. I have no pat answer. I volunteered for the county's AIDS project because I don't like the attitudes of some people. I'm a "buddy," which is basically a support person. We make meals, give baths, help people make funeral arrangements, and help them obtain legal counsel.

I'm involved because I believe in the best care possible for people irrespective of their lifestyle or socioeconomic status. That's why I work in a county institution. We refuse no one. I could never work in hospitals where patients are blatantly refused care because they cannot pay. I sure as hell am no saint—I get teed off at people regularly—but I can't justify denying anyone care. I couldn't live with myself.

PART THREE

NURSE SPECIALISTS

The power of expert knowledge brought to bear on difficult and complex patient situations is what nurse specialists are all about. Clinical nurse specialists tackle patient problems that the general nurse does not have the ability to solve. Nurse specialists gain their expert knowledge through master's education in areas of concentration such as neonatal care, critical care, child and family care, gerontology, or mental health.

Specialists may give care themselves, consult at the staff nurse's request, or guide staff in the direct care of the patient. Through their research, clinical specialists are originators in patient care methods. Quite often, their methods are as creative as they are clinical.

The five nurses in this section speak of the ways in which they handle particularly difficult nursing scenarios. In Jacqueline's case, the challenge of her duties is compounded by the fact that she is sightless. With the aid of her seeing-eye dog, Jacqueline offers expert counseling to chronically ill children and their families.

Catherine, a clinical specialist, also works with children, many of whom are frightened or angered by their physical prognoses. In one poignant example, Catherine tells of her work with a disturbed four-year-old burn victim, showing how the application of the growth and development theory can change a child's self-destructive behavior.

For Sara, the challenge of nursing isn't simply limited to her work with the developmentally disabled. In applying new care methods to these patients, Sara finds herself combatting a medical insurance system that places little value on her work. It involves a theme that repeats itself throughout this book: Healing the sick and mending the wounded offer encouraging statistics, while long-term care, with its uncertain, hard-to-pin-down results, can be expensive and frustrating. HMOs have only clouded the issues.

When push comes to shove, patients often need an informed, caring nurse to advocate for them. Susan, a clinical specialist in oncology nursing, specializes in bone marrow transplantation cases. It is a fairly new field in which results cannot always be accurately projected, and Susan tells how her work in this area has found her challenging doctors and nurse colleagues—all for the benefit of good patient care.

Nan, a mental health specialist is concerned with helping mentally ill patients express their anger constructively. Her main objective is to assist her patients in channeling self-destructive behavior. To save the lives of suicidal patients, she draws up contracts and literally gives new value to the phrase, "One day at a time."

The care given by these clinical specialists enhances the quality of life for those suffering from difficult illnesses. In some cases, the nursing care saves lives.

13

A Strong Will and a Strong Mind

Jacqueline White's cubicle office is tucked in the administrative wing of a children's hospital. As we enter, a German shepherd approaches us, sniffs, and then retreats, satisfied that we mean no harm.

"This is my dog, Owen," Jacqueline says, extending a hand. Her handshake is strong. "Owen is not only my eyes, but he's also like my child. As soon as he and I got together, it was love at first sight. We've been together ever since, going on nine years."

We sit down. The overhead light catches the golden highlights of Jacqueline's short-cropped hair. She is pretty and trim.

While we talk, it becomes apparent that Jacqueline, like any devoted nurse committed to a career of providing the best patient care possible, is a person who makes a difference.

I was lured into nursing through a combination of events. My first course in high school biology inaugurated me into the intricacies of the human body. I still think the human body is the most exquisite thing ever created. About that time, I was diagnosed as a diabetic. I was frequently in and out of the hopsital.

My experiences gave me a real understanding of what it's like to be a kid with a chronic illness. I can appreciate the pain, loneliness, fear, and lack of control that kids feel. I saw nursing as a way for me to help children. Pediatrics has been my consuming interest.

Immediately after obtaining my hospital school diploma, I went on to Temple University and received a bachelor's degree in nursing education. During that time, I worked in intensive care at St. Christopher's Hospital for Children in Philadelphia.

At this point, I was having severe trouble with my vision. I took time off for medical reasons—three years, to be exact. By then, I was legally blind, yet I knew I wanted to go to graduate school. I didn't know what it would be like to be blind and a student. I decided that I needed to carefully prepare for it if I were to be successful.

There are some tricks of the trade. Blind people need to learn to read by listening; they need to learn how to organize people to read to them. There's a variety of other skills people need to acquire to be successful as a blind student. All these can be done; it just takes time.

I enrolled at the University of Delaware and took courses through continuing education to master the skills I'd need in school as a blind student. When I knew I was ready, I applied and was accepted at Bryn Mawr, in the School of Social Work and Social Research. It was there I met Braulio Montalvo, a well-known family therapist. Braulio and I talked for hours. I decided to become a family therapist in order to work with families in a pediatrics hospital setting, and my discussions with Braulio helped to crystallize this plan.

While I was thinking about where to get my master's degree, I felt a real pull to return to nursing. Nursing was an essential part of my identity. I knew that if I failed to return to nursing, I'd regret it for the rest of my life.

How was it for me, to be blind and a graduate student in nursing? I was already blind when I was in the graduate program at Bryn Mawr. By the time I went to work on my master's at the University of Pennsylvania, it was fairly easy. The people in the nursing graduate program were pretty open-minded. It was a learning experience for everybody. I was the first blind student they'd had. They counted on me to give the faculty directions as to how I'd take notes and how I'd be taking exams. That sort of thing. Because I was blind, some learning techniques were unique, but it was not impossible. I obtained a master's in child and adolescent psychiatric nursing, with an emphasis on family therapy.

After I graduated from Penn, I went into private practice as a clinical nurse specialist. That was fine for a while, but I missed the collegial relationship, the support you get when you're working in an institution. I contacted children's hospitals to see if they'd hire a person to work exclusively with chronically ill children and their families. When I called the people here at Children's Hospital, the recruiter said, "You're just what we are looking for." I've been here two years now.

My job title is clinical nurse specialist for chronic illness. I explain to patients and staff that I am truly a child mental health specialist. It happens that, here at Children's Hospital, I concentrate my practice on children with chronic illnesses.

I work with the nursing staff as well as with the patients and families. I get referrals from both nurses and physicians. Most often, it is the staff nurse who calls me to see the child and family. The nurse may want me to consult with her about the patient, see the family, or actually take the patient on.

Recently, a staff nurse asked me to see the mother of a nine-year-old boy named Jeff. The mother was very upset about the procedures performed on her child. When I first saw the lady, she was crying uncontrollably. She could barely get the words out. Sure, the mother was angry about the procedures, but that wasn't the real problem. She was really grieving the loss of her healthy child. She'd taken him to the physician for what she thought was a bad cold, and suddenly she was told her robust child had a mysterious chronic lung ailment. She was overwhelmed.

The mother was unable to identify the real cause of her anger. I told her that it was natural for parents to be angry when they first learned of the diagnosis. This is part of the normal grieving process. We talked about a way to explain Jeff's illness to him in a nonfrightening way.

That was the beginning of my contact with this family. I've maintained this relationship to the present time. Jeff is home now. The mother calls me and asks questions like, "Should I discipline my son when he's been misbehaving? Is it safe for him to go to school? What should I tell my in-laws about what is wrong with Jeff?"

Another big concern this mother had—and that parents have, in general—is what to tell the brothers and sisters. There is no pat answer. First, I find out the ages of the children as well as what they know about illness and hospitals. For instance, have their friends ever been hospitalized? I encourage parents to explain the child's illness to his brother or sister. I tell the parents that parenting the sick child, in terms of setting limits, will be much the same as before he became ill, but he'll need to take care of himself differently. The difference will be that the child will need to take medications; he may need daily or weekly treatments; and from time to time he'll need to go to the hospital.

The parents also need to realize that their explanations to the siblings will change as they become older and when the sick child's condition alters. The first explanation is not the end, but only the beginning. As the child progresses developmentally, the questions will get tougher—"Will my brother or sister live?"—it doesn't get easier.

If I sense that a brother or sister is having a real rough time, I may see him or her. The siblings are individuals whose reactions will vary. I think it's universal that brothers and sisters think the sick child is getting more attention. Mom and Dad are spending lots of time away. The sick kids are getting lots of goodies and presents. At the same time, the siblings feel guilty that their brother or sister is ill. We encourage brothers or sisters to visit in the hospital and even help with the care of the child. They can smooth the blankets, get water, or play games.

Siblings want two roles. As with all normal children, they want to be different from their parents and counterparts—they want a special place within their families. At the same time, they want to be equal to their peers. Having a sibling with a chronic illness can stigmatize them; they become part of the family with "the diabetic child" or "the child with cystic fibrosis." Siblings don't like that.

Grandparents also react to the sick child. They, too, grieve for the loss of the healthy child. They play various roles. Some are not available, while others become the parenting experts. They are there to relieve the parents, to baby-sit for the other children.

There are the few grandparents who feel guilty, especially if the child has an inherited disease. They may blame themselves for "passing on" the disease, or you'll occasionally find a grandparent who takes sides or tries to lay blame for the inherited disease with comments such as, "My son or daughter couldn't be responsible for this."

This is just the nature of families. In those instances, I move in quickly to help them understand that blaming isn't helpful. Instead, we examine ways they can support each other. I try to reassure the child and parents that the child's chronic illness is not their fault, that these things happen.

I talk with the sick child about a number of things. First of all, I talk about what it is like to be in the hospital. That can be pretty scary. We talk about the food, the smells, the noises, and how hospitals are different from home. We discuss the scary things, such as Mom and Dad's not being there and the painful procedures. I tell them, "You may be mad when people poke you and hurt you. They'll ask you all kinds of strange questions."

When children get to know me, they talk about their fears. They hear a lot of strange words and they want to know what they mean. Take the case of this little girl, Susie, who was diagnosed as being diabetic. I checked with her parents to get their OK to explain her illness to her, and Susie and I talked about what it meant to have a chronic illness, about how it's something she'd learn to live with, that she could learn to live quite well with it. She could fly her kites, play with her dog, go to school. I touched upon the fact that she'd have to return to the hospital from time to time. This is a realistic part of having a chronic illness.

I see the children throughout their illnesses, even those who enter the terminal phase of their illnesses and enter the hospice program. I see them to the end. By following the child, I am saying to the child and family, "I can handle this and I can help you handle this."

I've found that children know they're going to die, but they don't say it outright. They let me know indirectly. Like little Joe, who said, "Gee, I'm worried that I need to be hospitalized more," or Timmy, the seven-year-old with cystic fibrosis who told me, "My breathing is harder," or Samantha who, when I asked her how things were going, said, "The medications aren't working like they used to—I need to use a wheelchair now."

Children grieve for themselves, for the loss of the person they were, for the loss of their health. Sometimes, they grieve in anticipation of their death. We tend to see this more with the older kids, the teenagers. They know what "terminal" is; they know what it means to say, "You have an illness with a shortened life expectancy." Some families are comfortable in sharing their pain, while some are not.

Sure, this work is stressful. I feel very sad when children are dying. I give myself permission to grieve. I have a few close friends with whom I commiserate. Everyone who works with children here needs a shoulder to cry on. Sometimes, I just get away, for a few hours or a day.

I guess it takes a certain kind of endurance. I mean that in a positive way. The fulfillment that I get from helping these people is greater than the sadness. Most families need temporary help to get them over the hump. I'm not here to hold their hands for the rest of their lives. I help them develop the skills needed to cope with the illness. I also realize that I can't fix every difficult situation. I wish I could, but I can't.

People react to my own physical disability in various ways. Children have a lot of questions. They'll say, "Gee, you have a dog. Why do you have a dog in the hospital?" Owen is warm and fuzzy and non-threatening, both to the kids and their parents. So I use him as an ice-breaker. The children can ask questions about my blindness through Owen, without feeling self-conscious. My dog acts as my co-therapist.

Some parents relate to my blindness as a loss similar to the one they are experiencing. Should they choose to do that, it's OK with me. I'm perfectly comfortable talking about what it meant to me to lose my vision in adulthood. If they don't make that connection, that's fine, because I have other things to offer in helping them come to terms with their child's illness.

Blindness is part of who I am, but it isn't *me.* My job is unique, not because I'm blind, but because most pediatric institutions do not have a nurse expert who cares exclusively for children with chronic illnesses and their families. All children's hospitals should have nurses with specialized knowledge of the emotional needs of chronically ill children and their families because a large portion of the patients in pediatric hospitals are children with chronic conditions.

It saddens me to hear that some nurses are dissatisfied and are leaving nursing. Nursing is a wonderful profession, from which I receive enormous satisfaction and fulfillment. To be sure, there are times when it is frustrating, when you are tired or what-have-you. But there are so many gratifying things that happen in a given week. There are numerous instances when I believe I have improved the quality of life.

I've been asked if a blind person could go through basic nursing programs. I've given it a lot of thought, and I think it's a pretty important question. I feel a responsibility when I'm asked that question because some blind person's potential career could be altered by my answer.

I'd have to initially say no. I think any person could do the course work, but I don't know how the person could function in the physical care of patients. Sure, the student without vision could give a bed bath. The student could even take a temperature with a braille thermometer. But could the individual detect circumoral cyanosis? No. So much nursing today is being able to read monitors. Could someone who is blind do that? No.

Sure, there are plenty of things you can do if you have gone through a generic program and then lose your sight. You've got the basic clinical experience to work from. When a staff person says, "The patient has circumoral cyanosis," you can conjure up a visual image. You remember what it looked like. It's almost impossible to explain "dusky" or "cyanosis" to a person who has been blind from birth and doesn't even know what color is.

14

Catherine's Added Difference

Dedicated clinical specialists glow when they describe their work with patients. When Catherine speaks of patient experiences, her eyes sparkle and her voice picks up a bright dimension.

In the past, I've considered other career alternatives, but even with all its problems, nursing is still the best career for me. Before I pursued my doctorate in educational psychology, my father encouraged me to think about medicine. "Be a pediatrician," he told me. "You'll make more money." He was right about the money, but medicine would have been too limiting for me.

In nursing, I can teach, do research in my area of interest, have patient and family contact. Working with children and families as I do gives me a special satisfaction. When a child is frightened, we nurses are there first to comfort. When a patient stops breathing, we are the first to initiate lifesaving measures. When a child dies, we are right there with the family, comforting them, holding them when they cry, crying with them.

Some people don't like to work with children; they say it takes too much patience. I seem to have a lot of patience with children, but not much with adults.

Children are so fascinating. They teach you about human nature. You see why adults are the way they are. The most rewarding part of caring for children is their tremendous courage. You see these little tykes—three, four years old—subjected to all this pain, suffering it better than any adult.

Teenagers are another courageous group. Here they are, being children, yet facing adult decisions. I recall a thirteen-year-old leukemic adolescent who eventually made the decision that she no longer would tolerate chemotherapy. In her case, the treatment was useless.

Another young leukemic, a sixteen-year-old black named Reggie, was so brave. He had claimed to be part of a gang. His family was very depressed, emotionally and socially. They were unable to support him through the dying process.

At first, he was acting out all over the place, not allowing anyone to help him. The psychiatrist saw him, talked with him, opened him up to his fears. Finally he said, "You mean I'm going to die?" The psychiatrist told him, "We are all going to die, Reggie, but you may die soon. We will help you if you let us." He started to cry—this big kid, half man, half child. After that, he didn't give in, but he let us help him in his own way. He didn't always ask for help, but he'd accept it.

I remember making patient rounds one day. Reggie was lying on the bed, staring into space, his TV blaring away. I told him I'd play a game of checkers with him if he wanted to. He nodded. A few minutes into the game, I noticed how weak he was. I said, "I know you're tired. How about if I just sit here with you? You talk if you want." He nodded. We just sat for a long time, maybe forty-five minutes, and he went off to sleep. He died that night.

I suppose the biggest influence on my career was a head nurse I knew during my student days in the hospital school. In those days, the head nurse was also the teacher. She gave the lectures, supervised the students, and ran the wards. This particular young woman was exceptional. She wore a hearing aid to compensate for a severe hearing loss sustained as a child.

She knew everything that had to do with the physical and psychological care of children. From her, I learned that nursing was more than carrying out the doctors' orders, or doing baths and treatments. I learned that nurses had a place helping patients and families adapt to their illnesses—we could be as strong as penicillin, so to speak.

She was very child oriented—before it was fashionable. In those days, many pediatric units really abused children. Limited visiting hours kept parents from their children at a time when the children needed them most. Some hospitals had the crazy practice of tying kids to the bed. Play was unheard of.

Not so on our unit. We encouraged parents to stay with their very sick kids, and we improvised beds so the parents could rest. Play was considered an important part of the youngster's recovery.

I recall a particular incident when the head nurse went to bat for her principles. I was playing with some kids who were immobilized due to traction and casts. Immobilization over a long period of time really causes youngsters to act out. It's a challenge to provide constructive ways for them to work off their excess energy. I had improvised a basketball game. The kids were throwing wads of paper at a wastebasket target. The winner was the person with the most wads of paper in the basket.

The supervisor came around and chastised me for playing and not working. She said that if that's all I had to do with my time she'd find a place where I could be used to give nursing care. The head nurse overheard and told her that I was acting on instructions from her, that I was doing nursing and play was an important part of children's care. The supervisor went off in a huff.

Today, play is considered an integral part of children's care. I use it in my practice all the time, as do my students. I use play to prepare a child for a procedure such as heart surgery, or for the playing out of other unpleasant experiences. It really is a wonderful therapy.

I recall a youngster who had ruptured his spleen in a car accident and had had the spleen removed. He was placed in intensive care for a few days following surgery. There were no signs of head injury, but the child seemed mute and wouldn't talk to the staff or his parents. We brought out a hospital play kit, containing equipment used on children, such as stethoscopes, flashlights, blood pressure cuffs, and so on. We started to play, and he quickly joined in.

In intensive care, a flashlight was used to check his pupil reaction, and this seemed to bother him. He grabbed the flashlight from the kit and flashed it into a doll's eyes, repeating the procedure for most of the play sessions. He then used the other equipment on the doll. Within a few days, he was talking to beat the band. Most childhood illnesses have an emotional component. Children's fear and insecurity is often expressed by their physical behavior. Emotional problems may cause physical illnesses like anorexia. Or the physical illness can result in an emotional reaction.

As a clinical specialist, I try to anticipate what the children's needs may be, in order to prevent complications. I do this by meeting with staff, helping them to plan care, or I may take care of the child myself. It is usually a team effort, especially in complex situations. Sometimes the patient is too much for the staff to handle and they call me in.

Lots of children I've cared for have been very special to me, but there are always the few you will never forget. It's been quite a while, but I can still remember a little four-year-old with second- and third-degree burns. The head nurse asked me to see Lisa because the staff could no longer cope with her self-destructive behavior.

Lisa had been admitted some six weeks earlier with burns. A pot of boiling water had toppled over the side of a kitchen stove, spilling the steaming liquid over her neck and chest. I can still visualize the way she looked the first time I saw her. She was lying on her back, the fingers of her right hand busy picking the skin from her left wrist. At the time, silver nitrate dressings were used on burns. When the time was right, grafting followed. The silver nitrate discolored the surrounding intact tissue, giving it a grayish appearance. The skin became dried and cracked. This change in her body image frightened Lisa. She frantically picked at her skin, trying to uncover the original color. The result was patches of raw, oozing red body surfaces. Though her hands were restrained, she quickly learned to maneuver her way out of the gauze bindings. During fits of temper, she would pull her hair out. This resulted in stark, bald areas from the mid-line of her head to her ears.

At her bedside, hanging from a pole, was a quart bottle of dark liquid. It flowed through a tube through her nose to her stomach. Since she refused food, the supplement provided the nourishment she needed for survival. There was a stink to the room, coming from Lisa's involuntary bowel movement. She no longer had control of her bowel or bladder.

Unlike the other children, who had many visitors in and out during the day, Lisa had visitors only on occasional weekends. Lisa's family lived two hundred miles from the hospital. Her mother had been with her during the first week of hospitalization. However, she was in her ninth month of pregnancy, and she returned home to care for her other children and await the birth of her eighth child.

If you didn't understand the reasons for Lisa's behavior, you'd imagine she was unbalanced. In nursing, we say, "Put yourself in the patient's place." Since we all have been children, pediatrics is one place you can do this.

Do you remember being told, as a child, to stop being naughty or something bad would happen to you? When a four-year-old has had an accident like Lisa's burns, she can only think it's because she'd been bad. The burn therapy itself hurts like hell. There is no way to say to a four-year-old, "I know this hurts, but it's for your own good." You just have to find other ways to let her know that you like her and are sorry you hurt her.

Being in a strange place, separated from your mom, is scary. Do you recall how you felt as a child when you got separated from your mom, say, in the grocery or department store? Now put this all together. You hurt so bad. You don't know why your mom had to leave you when you need her so much. She'd always been there for you before. To top it off, she's left you with strangers who hurt you unbearably, who tell you they're doing it for your own good.

The only conclusion a four-year-old can reach is that she is bad and nobody loves her. She reasons, "They couldn't love me and do this to me." The hatred can turn inward, and you get bizarre happenings, such as kids' pulling their hair out.

I remember being overwhelmed at the state Lisa was in. I made a plan of care and consulted the child psychiatrist. He thought my ideas were on the right track, and he encouraged me to go ahead with my plan. My knowledge of growth and development told me that this child needed intense mothering. I knew that if she was to trust me, I'd need to be fairly visible. I would go and take care of her several hours every day—even on weekends, for several weeks. I needed to work like this at first. There are no regular hours to a job like this; you come and go, according to the patient's needs.

At first, I concentrated on taking care of her body. I'd do the things a mother would do. I bathed her, rubbed her with lotion. I tried to reinforce the idea that I thought she was pretty by fixing her up, putting ribbons in her hair, telling her how pretty she was. I encouraged others to do so, especially the men to whom she responded well. It was obvious that she had been mothered well, as she responded to comforting and touching. She was still too weak to walk. I'd hold her in my lap, rock her, and sing to her.

Every afternoon, I put her to sleep. I'd sit at the bedside and stroke her forehead and sing to her. At first, she was fretful and slept for short periods. Eventually, her sleep became long and restful. One day, I decided to test out if my care made a difference in her sleep. I drew the shades and told her that it was nap time. I just sat at the side of the bed and didn't touch her. A few minutes went by. She opened her eyes and said angrily, "Hey, you aren't helping me to get to sleep at all."

"I'm sorry," I said, and I began to stroke her forehead. Within minutes, she was deep in sleep.

Her appetite was so poor that I catered to her food wants with hot dogs, french fries, and ice cream. When she felt better about herself, her appetite improved.

Lisa needed to know that someone in the strange environment would protect her. I took on the role of the "good nurse." That is, I wouldn't administer the painful treatments. Every day, she was placed in a tub and her burns were gently scrubbed with gauze. I made sure she received pain medication well in advance of the therapy. Still, the pain was excruciating. I would comfort her and hold her after the treatments.

Once she knew she had an ally, she stopped pulling her hair out and picking at her skin. I told her I didn't want her to do it, that I liked her too much to let her hurt herself. I told her I knew she was mad, but she didn't need to hurt herself—she was a good girl. She could get her "mad" out in other ways. I got darts that she could throw from her bed to a board mounted on the wall.

Kids this age like to control. We allowed her to control her therapy wherever we could. The feeding tube needed to be changed periodically. The hospital policy only allowed physicians to change tubes. I taught Lisa to change her own. The doctors were very cooperative; I had them come to the doorway and look on. Lisa pretended the tube was a sword and she was the sword swallower. This way, she passed the tube by herself; otherwise, we would have needed to hold her down. I still chuckle when I think about it—administration never knew anything about our breach of policy. Sometimes, nurses need to go around policy and we knew it was safe to do so with Lisa.

When the grafts on her legs healed, she was able to get out of bed. She was able to play more vigorously and use play to safely get out her feelings. We used water play. We gave her some dolls, and she named each doll after a staff member. She'd place the dolls in the water. She'd fill a water gun and squirt the water at the dolls, killing off the staff, one by one. She really couldn't understand the reason staff had to hurt her. Killing us off in play allowed her a healthy way to get out her anger without alienating those upon whom she also depended.

Her mother loved her very much, but the child didn't know this. All the pain and loneliness got distorted. She felt rejected. I recall the day I was reading her the story of *Black Beauty.* We were at the part where the stable boy blames himself because he neglected to rub the horse down and Black Beauty got pneumonia. Suddenly, Lisa started to cry, saying, "It wasn't my fault I got burned."

"Of course it wasn't your fault," I told her. "You're a good girl, and your mother and father love you very much. They are waiting for you to get home."

She responded with a vehemence greater than I realized a four-year-old could have. "You don't know nothin'," she said. "There's no room at home, no room for me to sleep."

As we talked, I realized that she thought the new baby would take her place in the already crowded bed. There would be no room for her.

Lisa had been placed in isolation to protect her from hospital infections, so she couldn't leave the room to call home. We wrote letters to her parents and siblings. I called her mother and encouraged her to have the family visit and, if possible, bring pictures. Remember, the family lived two hundred miles away and these people were poor.

They managed to come. I asked Lisa how her visit went. She showed me some pictures of her brothers and sisters, and she looked at me with her big eyes. "Know what?" She looked like she was bursting to tell a secret.

"What?" I asked.

"Ma says to hurry and get better, 'cause they're waiting for me at home," she replied.

15

Catching Up

Seventeen years ago, Sara graduated from the first graduate program for family and child clinical specialists. Her entire career has been devoted to the special needs of developmentally delayed.

Working with the developmentally delayed has been my whole life. I went to school, to get my master's degree in nursing, with a heavy emphasis on growth and development, and I came back here to the Children's Hospital to start the intervention clinic. I work with a physician and social worker, and we have a team approach.

During my career, I've developed my own practice techniques, since there were none available when I started. For example, I created my own developmental interviews. Initially, I plot where my patients are, in comparison to normal children; then we work with them to catch up to the next step. Catching up is a long, involved process. There are thirty-six movements just in eating. I look to see where the child is in this process and try to determine how we can get him to move ahead. The same applies to other activities of daily living. I've had a developmentally delayed child actually walk at fourteen months, another toilet trained at twenty months. That's quite a feat.

Over the years, I've developed some unique tools for the children, such as special spoons for eating, special kinds of kick boards to help in the development of their lower limbs.

Our philosophy in the intervention clinic is that parents are the best teachers. It really makes sense that the new baby be kept at home, and we try to teach the parents to learn the special techniques necessary to parent the child with developmental disabilities. Some programs for developmentally delayed children have two-month-olds bused to a center for active stimulation. From my observation, this isn't as effective. The bond between the parent and child is itself a stimulus for the child to achieve. That, coupled with certain activities, really works wonders.

I see the children regularly, up to eighteen months; then they are referred to places like Easter Seals services, which do respite care for parents. Regular baby-sitters, for example, are leery of sitting for developmentally delayed children; Easter Seals provides baby-sitters for a small fee.

Though I see parents only during a child's infancy, the parents have kept in touch with me over the years. I guess it's because they are so desperately in need of someone when they first hear the child has a developmental disability. I help them during their grief and see them through. A special bond forms. It's great to see how well some of these kids do later on.

I've kept in touch with Sammy, a Down syndrome child who is doing very well. He's school age and sings "Frère Jacques" in French. He tells me, "Quiet, Sara, sit down and listen to me," and then he goes on to sing. It's those kinds of things that make twelve-hour days worthwhile.

Physicians directly refer the kids to me. They know now, after all this time, what I can do. Parents also refer other parents to me. However, in order for me to be reimbursed for the referral, a physician must write the order for the care that I give.

Now, with Health Maintenance Organizations, we are having some real problems in maintaining our program. The child must be referred to personnel within the particular HMO to which his parents belong. The problem is some HMOs have no one who has the special skills necessary to work with these kids. I have HMO nurses calling me to say that they're going out to these kids and they have never even taken care of a *baby* since training, let alone a developmentally delayed youngster. It's getting bad for us financially. All we have coming in is some state subsidy—that, plus whatever the parents might have from insurance, covers our cost. Due to the HMOs, the insurance coverage is not available. I don't know what will happen to our program in the future.

One of our mothers just testified at the state hearings on problems in accessing care in some of the HMOs. She talked about the inferior care. One HMO wouldn't pay for her child's braces because braces weren't in the reimbursement policies. She fought this ruling and finally got the braces, though she claimed they were of inferior quality and broke very quickly.

What is depressing is that work with developmentally delayed children is no longer valued. We know that early intervention makes a tremendous difference in the long-term outcome of these kids. I hope things turn around.

16

The Advocate

Transplantation of bone marrow from a healthy person to an afflicted person helps prolong life in certain types of leukemia, anemia, and immune deficiencies. Transplant patients have complex medical regimens that require close supervision by both physicians and nurse specialists. Susan is a clinical specialist in oncology nursing: the nursing of people with cancer.

I've been in oncology since 1970. My work as a clinical specialist is to assess what needs to be done for the oncology patients and decide how well staff are prepared to do these things. I teach the nurses how to do the specialized care routines. I deal with quality issues. For example, why we are doing our I.V. therapy a certain way—is there a better way? It's a constant evaluation process. My role differs from the physician's in that the physician's primary role is to offer options for curative or management intent to the patient.

In my role, I do some of the patient physical assessments that physicians do, but I do them for nursing reasons. I may ask, "Based on past experiences, what does this current illness mean to the patient?" I do a lot of patient teaching. It's important that the patient know what to do for himself at home. We can carry out the care regimen in the hospital, but who will do it at home?

I translate to a patient what a physician is saying, and I discuss with the patient what the diagnosis and treatment will mean for him. We do a lot more translating and spend more time with patients than anyone else on the health team. I do believe that doctors sometimes talk deliberately above the patient's level of comprehension, which is confusing. If the patient doesn't have any idea what the doctor is talking about, he isn't likely to ask him questions.

As a clinical specialist, I identify patient problems and research ways to alleviate or minimize them. I'm now studying ways to lessen nausea and vomiting for patients receiving chemotherapy. This is particularly important because some people get so sick from the therapy that they wonder if they should quit and not come back to the hospital.

Some practitioners think drugs are the only answer for nausea, but they don't use them properly. I'm studying ways to make anti-emetic drugs more effective. I'm also looking for ways to decrease nausea without using drugs. We found that lying flat increases nausea, so we removed the examining tables from the clinic area and have only chairs for outpatient treatments. This has made a real difference in decreasing nausea and vomiting. The nurse is the one to research these things. My advanced education has helped me be able to identify such problems and study them. I wouldn't know how to conduct research without my master's degree.

I've never been so emotionally depleted that I felt I wanted to stop nursing cancer patients. *They* aren't the problem—the *system* is. The number one problem in being a clinical specialist is lack of appreciation by the nurses you work with, superiors and peers. The power plays of the physicians, and how they try to pit the nurses against each other, is also a problem. Even when you have established a good working relationship with physicians, they seem to do things to protect themselves or get the better end of the deal. It's an endless power struggle.

For example, when the physicians recently found out that we were going to begin charging for our nursing services, they threatened to bring in physicians' assistants to take our place. That way, the physicians would indirectly get the money we would be working for. We may have won that battle, but I'm disappointed by what I thought was a really good working relationship.

I still worry that we nurses may not be strong enough to win our case again, if the physicians should decide that they really need that money. I wonder, too, if nursing administration would back us up, or if the hospital administration would give in to the physicians in order to get something else they need more.

The physicians get frustrated with the system over which they also have little control. Maybe things get delayed because, say, the clerks only work at their own pace. The clerks are unionized, so you can't do much with them. Anyway, the doctor gets mad at the slowdown and blames the nurses for foul-ups in the system. They threaten to bring in physician's assistants so they can have the same kind of control they have in private practice offices. This produces real frustrations. The doctors do have a point—the system should change so *all* of us can deliver better care to patients.

We started a bone marrow unit before we were ready. We should have had policies and procedures in place before we opened, but nursing at a high level was involved in the decision to start the unit early. The head physician was very aggressive, and he wanted the unit started. I was the only nurse who protested the early start. I did so because I knew we weren't organized for care. I knew we'd have staffing and patient problems. But the old guilt trip was laid on us—"All those patients are out there, ready for transplants, and they may die if you don't do them." Well, hell, there must be other places nearby that are doing transplants successfully. The bottom line was money. We doubled the hospital income with our unit, and we didn't have to hire other people.

It went fairly well at first. We had a small, cohesive work group. Then we drew other people in. They started to question our policies because they'd been hastily put together. The head physician wasn't around much, so I had no support for ironing out problems in a very new program. Higher physician visibility would have given greater credibility to what we were doing, but no one was really giving directions.

A bigger frustration is lack of appreciation from the staff nurses I work with. Staff nurses on the unit feel frustrated themselves, and then they dump on me. I got in there to make sure things got off to a good start for the bone transplant patients, but I'm now abused. The unit nurses expect me to consistently work overtime. I'm willing to help out, but sometimes their demands get to be too much. I value my specific role as a clinical specialist. The unit will go on, with or without my support. If I'm always filling in on the oncology unit, my own work won't get done. I need to decide what I can do that others can't do and let the staff nurses do their own day-to-day nursing.

The staff nurses should complain to nursing administration about the fact that they were working harder without extra help. There is a lot of back-biting on the unit. It's really because they don't know how to be assertive; instead, they're aggressive or confrontational in a non-problem-solving way.

My experience in my last job was much different. The philosophy was different. Nurses were more assertive because they knew nursing administration would always back them up. Here, you can't count on the support of nursing administration.

Would you believe that, this last weekend, a physician demanded that the bone marrow transplant nurses staff the intensive care unit? See, some bone marrow patients may go to intensive care after the transplant. Since when does a physician tell nurses how to do their staffing? Nursing administration went along with it, and the physician got his way. All weekend, the oncology unit was seriously understaffed. They weren't looking at what pulling unit staff into intensive care would do to the quality of care on the unit or to staff morale.

Of course, in any relationship, one has to estabish trust in the other. We need to trust doctors, and they need to trust us. It's different in the clinic. The staff physicians know us and have worked extensively without misuse of nurses.

When I intervene there with patients, my judgments are trusted. I can work up a patient who has a temperature in outpatient, treat him, and send him home—and *then* communicate these treatments to the physician. The medical house staff aren't nearly that assured about nurses' decisions because we haven't established our credibility with each other.

I remember helping a young nurse deal with her own bone cancer. She wanted to be a code—that is, to receive life-support measures if she stopped breathing. She was receiving morphine for pain through a continuous intravenous drip. Our current nursing policy stated that a patient couldn't have a morphine drip unless she was a no-code. When the staff found out she was a code, they discontinued the drip. They attempted to talk her into a no-code so they could start the morphine drip again. It was like saying, "We'll take care of you and give you pain medications only if you'll agree to die." I talked to the supervisor and we changed the policy. The lady went home with a morphine drip and died at home.

I felt good about helping to change that policy. Who are *we* to make these decisions about others? So much goes into a patient's decision. Who are *we* to negate their past histories? It's their decision, as long as they are as fully informed as we can help a patient to be. I may be in the same situation someday, and that's the way I would like to be treated.

I'm not always popular for my stand as a patient advocate. Not so long ago we had a Mexican patient dying. When Mexicans die, the whole family comes to pay their respects. There must have been more than forty people in the room. The staff said only three could be in the room at one time. Well, why not let them in the patient's room, as long as they aren't obstructing other patients' rights? I worked fifteen hours that day because I knew he would die and I was afraid there would be problems. I said that the family could stay. Some of my staff were very angry with me, and they're probably still angry, but I can take it. I can live with it. I'm here for the patient, not to win a popularity contest.

I try to remember that someone has to consider the idea that the patient and family have special needs. I can only hope that someone will do the same for me someday.

17

New Age Nurse

We are sitting in Nan's office, which is located at the end of the patients' care unit. Pink chintz curtains adorn the windows. Nan sits in her "thinking" position: shoes off, feet propped up on a cushioned stool, a stuffed pillow hugged to her bosom. Utterly relaxed, Nan relates her contributions to people's mental health.

I have a master's degree and certification as a mental health specialist through the American Nurses' Association. I left oncology for mental health. In oncology, I had little old men from West Texas who avoided talking about things they didn't want to talk about, and not talking about these things was contributing to their illnesses. But I discovered that over a game of dominos they'd start to talk about the lymph angiogram [X-ray of lymph vessels] and how badly it scared them.

I opted to work a summer in psychiatry in order to improve my interviewing skills. I learned to help people who were experiencing emotional pain. I found I had an ability to walk in another person's shoes—understand how they were feeling—and still be in my own shoes. What happens to us, when we become scared and see no outlet, is tunnel vision. That's true of anyone, whether you're a patient or a member of a staff. My role is to say, "Let's examine your problem in a different way."

In my job, I function according to the classical description of the clinical nurse specialist. I am a researcher, consultant, teacher, and clinician. As teacher, I pass my clinical skills on to others. For example, when I taught in Texas, one of my students cared for a man with terminal cancer of the lung. He was very angry and acted out. He'd made his wife and family so angry with him that they refused to visit. I taught the student several techniques for helping the man express his anger constructively. Before the man died, he was able to see his family and mend fences with them. In the end, he said he was looking forward to death and the beautiful place he was going to.

The unit I'm on is unique. We accept psychiatric patients who also have medical problems. We take cardiac and home dialysis patients who have been referred to us because they've developed severe depression. A traditional unit would have difficulty handling the mental problems of these patients. I direct patient care here, either with the individual or a group.

We work as a team, headed by a psychiatrist. There is also an internist, psychologist, social worker, dietician, recreational therapist, and occupational therapist. We meet three times a week to review the patients and coordinate their care. No single discipline is responsible for the evolution of the patient's care. We all contribute.

My input to the team varies. Sometimes I play the meanie. I ask the questions that the team members may be avoiding, such as "What secondary gain is this patient seeking?" In other words, how is this behavior serving the patient? What would he lose if he gave up the behavior? How are we helping or not helping this patient to keep his inappropriate behavior?

I've found, through study and my own ten years of experience, that we often do things unwittingly, to keep patients from changing their behavior. For example, take a patient who is depressed and takes to his bed. If we don't do anything about getting him up, how are we feeling about ourselves and our ability to help him move? Why do we allow him to continue his depressive behavior? The psychiatrist or social worker see the patient for a short time

—they lack the perspective. Most of the nurses on the unit don't have the advanced education, or the long-term experience, that is necessary to pick up those cues.

So my role is to create a different kind of a bridge between the patient situation and the team's observations. All of the team members come with a medical background as well as one in psychiatry, and we all ask the same major questions—"How much of the patient's problem is physical, and how much is due to his efforts to protect himself from the pain he'd have to endure regarding something else going on in his life?"

I tend not to see people as having a lot of pathology. I tend to see them as having a lot of emotional pain and coping with it as best they can. It's different from the medical approach, which views the patient's behavior as pathological. A lot of nurses also lean toward the medical viewpoint.

I, too, know the diagnostic classifications, but first I ask myself, "What's frightening this client?" I ask the client, "If you weren't having that severe backache, what would come in your mind? How is your backache protecting you from facing up to something else?"

I once had a patient who had a tremendous amount of trauma in her life—major sexual assaults as a child. She was severely abused in her marriage, and she focused on physical complaints. She was highly upset when she was first admitted because she didn't have a private room. Even knowing that we had no private room to give her, she yelled for over forty-five minutes that she would only take a private room.

The staff got upset. They continued to explain the fact that there was no private room. I finally said, "Wait a minute. She knows there is no private room. Something else is bothering her."

I went to the patient and said, "You know there is no private room. If you weren't focusing on the bed situation, what would you have to focus on?"

She said, "I'd have to focus on how angry I am with my first husband."

I said, "Fine. Let's talk about that. Talking about a single room that isn't available isn't getting us anywhere. Let's start to look at your anger toward your former husband."

It helps all of us to learn the message beneath the message. It's scary to confront what's really bothering us. Sometimes I'm really scared to look at my own problems because they hurt so bad the first time around that I think I'd die if I had to think of them again. But the reality is I survived those terrible experiences, whatever they were. The memory only has the power to hurt me if I'm not willing to face it.

A woman by the name of Lynn Andrews once wrote, "The things in our lives which control us are the things at which we refuse to look." I personally know the problems I created for myself because I wasn't willing to look at the anger I had toward my father. When I got into nursing school I was considered a good student but one heck of a troublemaker. The instructors would say, "Yeah, that Nan, she's really good, but when she gets up on a soapbox, look out, 'cause she's really trouble."

The reality was, when one of my instructors got dogmatic, like my dad, that person got the anger that was intended for my dad. I worked on issues about my dad in my own therapy.

See, as little children, we decide how important we are or aren't. When I was three and my mom was sick, I decided that I'd have to take care of myself. That made me fiercely independent, but that also kept me from allowing people to help me out. Then I'd get angry because no one would help me, even though I wouldn't let them.

If I asked you to go out on the street and ask a three-year-old how she wanted to manage her life, you'd think I'd lost my mind. Yet we let the three-year-old we used to be run our lives.

Therapy lets people go back and check out their childhood decisions and decide whether they still want to keep them. If a decision has kept things working well, terrific. Keep it. If it hasn't, what do we want to base our present reality on?

So I spend a lot of time with people, looking at old issues. Therapy is not placing blame on moms and dads; it's for looking at how old experiences affect our lives now. Do they help or hinder us? None of us can change our past, but we don't need to let the past dictate the present.

It's exciting to see people change. I followed a client, a self-mutilator, for several years. She'd been in the hospital nearly fifteen months when her primary therapist suggested that I also work with her. Mabel kept a razor blade in her car, so she could cut herself whenever the urge hit her. She also kept a bottle of aspirins, even though she knew she was allergic to them and could die from an anaphylactic reaction if she took them. If she decided that she absolutely had to die right then, she could eat the aspirin in the car and kill herself on the freeway.

Her birthday gift to me last year was the razor blade from her car. In spite of many recent crises in her life, she has only cut herself twice in the last six years—a significant gain from daily nicks at her body. She still has episodes where she thinks she is going crazy, but they don't debilitate her to the extent that she needs hospitalization. Instead of enduring depression for several months, her episodes of depression now last only a few days.

My instant rewards come from the little things. The patient who comes to therapy, even though he'd canceled numerous times before; the patient who can finally hold eye contact and sit, when all he could do before was pace; the patient who first comes into my office saying he feels numb and then is able to release his emotions and cry. These baby steps eventually lead to huge leaps.

Most people who have been abused emotionally or physically run away from themselves and avoid their thoughts. I try to get these people to stay present with themselves so they do not re-create past fears and angers. Naturally, they will experience new pain. Pain is part of living. But do they accept emotional pain as a sign that they're alive and growing, or is it something that immobilizes them?

I have them consider life events similar to a ride on a rollercoaster: When you come over the top, are you scared or excited? If you're excited, it's so much more fun. When you're over the top, you know you've accomplished a feat.

If you're scared, you never appreciate the thrill of accomplishment.

A lot of people I see have retreated from life. If they can learn to handle life, no one else will have to tell them how to do it. They come to know that they are the experts on themselves. This process doesn't happen overnight. There are no pat answers. In fact, I buried the "Book of Right Answers." If we always look for right answers, we never get anything done.

There is no one way to help people like themselves better, gain a greater variety of coping skills, or to take charge of their lives and their relationships. I'm an eclectic—I use whatever works. I may use an analytical model or psych assessment, a developmental approach, or a rational emotive technique. I may use transactional analysis to explain things to a patient. I may blend Eastern thought with Western medicine, work through the mind-body connections using Reiki body work techniques.

Many of us are out of touch with our own bodies. We don't communicate between our heads and the rest of us. Body work deals with the energy fields around the body; it's a way of helping people access their emotions more effectively. I can't explain how it works. I only know that it does.

A woman came into my office who had recently had a hysterectomy. She'd had a lot of grief over the loss of her uterus because she'd lost the dream of ever giving birth to her own child. Sitting near her, I could feel a tremendous amount of heat even though her oral temperature was normal. She wanted to cry, but she wasn't able to. You could see how her loss was causing her emotional pain.

She complained of continued physical pain, even though there was no physical reason. I asked her permission to touch her. I laid a hand on her chest, the other on her abdomen over the incisional area. A few minutes later, she exclaimed, "What are you doing? It's helping the pain!" Then the tears started to flow.

Thank goodness I'm a nurse. It gives me permission to use touch. Psychologists today are having difficulty with touch due to all the recent publicity about sexual abuse of patients. I always ask my patients' permission to touch them. I am concerned, at times, that someone will misinterpret the touch. Most clients give permission. Patients expect nurses to touch them.

Therapeutic touch is fascinating. When I scan over pain areas, I can feel the blockage of energy over the area. Placing my hand strategically on the area makes a difference. It's as if the energy from my hand flows to the pained area and the pain is relieved.

Now, I'm talking about bodily perception of psychic pain, such as the pain this lady had. Of course, she couldn't differentiate the pain source. The physical pain was very real to her. After she was able to cry, the physical pain was gone and she felt better emotionally.

Try this when you want to cry and can't. Hold your breath. It increases the chest tension and it hurts; it increases pressure in your head and it hurts, too. My patients laugh at me. They'll say, "I know, 'Keep breathing.' " It's fun, and they get playful with it. It's something taken from Eastern yoga that all of us can do. I use whatever works.

I sometimes use imagery mixed with whatever medical mores or belief systems the client has. One of the clients I worked with had what she believed to be experiences with a Satanic cult. She believed she saw spirits and other things and that there were other parts of the universe to which those spirits could be sent.

I had her imaging those spirits as being encased in a white light and taken to another part of the universe until they had healed and didn't need to be mean anymore. That image fit into her belief system and it worked. The evil spirits departed.

Sometimes imagery can be used to create a place where a person cannot be frightened. I help them to visually make that place real. They'll imagine a safe nook in some part of the house, full of stuffed animals and storybooks. Imaging a peaceful area helps people to become enmeshed in that place and let go of the pain. It is a wonderful adjunct to pain medication.

In short-term pain situations, such as during a bone marrow biopsy, I use contralateral applications of ice. Placing ice on the opposite hip helps to diminish the hip pain on the biopsy site.

People with phobias can use imagery in anxiety-producing situations. I have them mentally practice successfully getting through a frightening situation. It's pretty much like training an athlete—if you watch track stars on TV, you'll see them rehearse before they jump. If a client is afraid to go to a meeting, I'll have him visualize the meeting. What will it look like? What will people wear? Is the room smoky? They'll clearly repeat whatever it is that they will have to say or do for successful accomplishment.

Most of us are uncomfortable accepting our own responsibility for things that happen. It's easier to look at others and blame them for our problems. "I'm a victim, helpless and innocent," we say. In reality, we're not innocent. We may have set things up to look that way, but we've contributed. We may not feel particularly good as victims, but it got us off the hook, saved us from having to take responsibility for our behavior.

Mental health professionals can be blind to their own mental problems. I frequently check how honest I'm being with myself. I have to have good mental health if I'm going to avoid confusing my stuff with the client's. When a patient comes into my office looking real sad, it's important for me to know that it's *his* sadness and not mine.

My consultation with the other units in the hospital is just starting. Nursing staff have me assess their suicidal patients to determine if they need a sitter for constant surveillance. A sitter costs the hospital around twenty-five dollars an hour.

My job is to interview the patient to determine if he's really suicidal. Will he make another attempt? I'll ask outright, "Do you plan to kill yourself?" You need to believe what the patient answers. Most people you interview are relieved when you say, "Tell me about your pain. Sounds like you are hurting incredibly. Do you want to be dead? Do you want to stop the hurt?" The person is able to make a contract to postpone suicide. If you really want to kill yourself, nobody can really prevent you from doing so.

I don't ask people to give up suicide. I only ask that they postpone their suicide until we can look at what other alternatives would relieve their emotional pain. We make a contract, for say eight hours, that they won't try anything. Then the team works on ways for them to deal with their emotional pain. At the end of the eight hours, we renegotiate.

If they can maintain the contract longer, fine. Some people will say, "I really want to be dead, but I won't do it in the hospital." People who can't make any contract at all are definitely people who are at high risk to make another attempt. They may have already figured out how to kill themselves in the hospital. For sure, we will not leave that person without someone there with them at all times. I teach the nurses how to deal with the patients between the contract periods.

On the surgical units, I review drug therapy for any patient who has a psych problem and has had an operation. I help the nurse to know how the drugs work, what the safe parameters are for giving medications, what symptoms will tell you the patient has had too much.

Nurses tend to be very judicious in giving narcotics and other drugs. Sometimes, psychotropic drugs should be given as often as every hour to people who are hallucinating. The surgical nurse will look at the order and say, "My God, I can't give that much drug; the patient will overdose." With severe hallucinations, the patient may need the drug that frequently or he becomes terrified and very inappropriate. That happened last week—a patient got wired and hit a nurse.

It's terrifying to patients to be out of control, to be floridly psychotic. If the nursing and medical staff aren't aggressive enough getting the patient back in control, the patient thinks, "My God, even the people who are supposed to know how to get me back in control can't do it. I must be even worse off than I thought." So the person gets even more out of control.

The nursing staff on the general floors really want to take good care of these patients; it's just that they haven't had experience with these types of patients. They'll even stop me in the cafeteria to ask for advice.

I enjoy teaching staff. I'd be a damn fool, though, if I said that I don't get something extra special out of being a nurse. Some people say, "You're so altruistic." That's garbage. I do this because I get a lot out of it. It's important that the patient grows, too. It needs to be a win-win—every time.

PART FOUR

FILLING THE GAPS

The Surgeon General's Report of the 1960s predicted that large populations of the U.S. would not have access to health care to which they were entitled. An outgrowth of this dire prediction was a scramble by DHEW to develop a cadre of health workers who could extend medical care under the supervision of a physician. Nurse educators used this opportunity to train nurse practitioners. These nurses, like physicians, were trained to provide health screening as well as to diagnose and treat minor illnesses. Many went beyond the medical tasks to institute programs of wellness and prevention.

A December 1986 report of the U.S. Government Office of Technical Assessment concluded, after an intensive study, that "Nurse practitioners and midwives have the potential to reduce health care costs," and that "Nurse practitioners are more effective than physicians in the management of chronically ill patients." Similarly, the study stated that certified nurse midwives could manage normal pregnancy as well as, if not better than, physicians. According to the government report, the average salary of the nurse midwife was 25 percent of that of the physician/obstetrician.

This section describes the less costly, quality alternative that nurse practitioners, midwives, and anesthetists are safely offering to the people of this nation. The four nurses presented, though dependent by law on doctors' supervision, offer alternatives to standard medical services.

Ruth, the director of the New York City Maternity Center, offers data that proves that nurse midwives reduce morbidity and mortality rates for infants and mothers while providing a less expensive alternative to traditional hospital deliveries. Tessie, manager of a kidney transplant follow-up clinic, is an assertive patient care coordinator who often has to go to bat for her patients. The same can be said of Sister Monica, a Franciscan nun and registered nurse, who talks of her experiences with running a health care clinic serving the inner city's indigent. Ross, a nurse anesthetist, talks of the ways his nursing skills offer a less expensive alternative to the services afforded by anesthesiologists. Taken together, these four voices offer hints about possible nursing directions to be taken in the future, as well as the frustrations that will greet them.

18

The Plight of Midwives

Ruth's salt-and-pepper hair, conservative dark blue suit, and matronly reserve do not reflect the true woman. Indeed, she has been the recipient of honorary doctorates from prestigious universities and is a relentless champion for the rights of women. Her speech is slow and deliberate, honed by hours of testifying at congressional hearings on midwifery.

The Maternity Center Association of New York has been around since 1917 and has been nurse-run except for the first few years, when Francis Perkins was its director. The New York Maternity Center grew out of an agency project of the Women's City Club in New York. It was an outgrowth of the charitable work of women at the time. The agency established the first school of nurse midwifery. It has always conducted parent education classes. In the twenties, we tried to set up a midwifery direct-entry program, but it didn't work. For one reason, the physicians didn't want it; they were busy trying to eliminate midwifery because many of the midwives coming to this country were illiterate. Even when we became educated, their old biases against midwives persisted.

In 1931, the first school of nurse midwifery was established here in New York City, using public health nurses and offering an eight-month program. It established a home birth service for women in Central and East Harlem. Some pregnant women were afraid of hospitals; we worked to get them into hospitals.

The Maternity Center Association has a board of directors which is made up of consumers, not health professionals. The board gives total responsibility for the program to me. We have a board of physicians which is only advisory, but whose advice is always respected. Sometimes the board of directors accepts the physicians' advice, and sometimes it doesn't. However, the physicians' board serves to legitimize the center to the physician community. It's always more effective to get a physician to change another physician's attitudes.

It wasn't until 1971 that physicians of the American College of Obstetrics and Gynecology finally recognized nurse midwifery. I'm fond of saying we wandered in the wilderness for over forty years. Nationally, by that time there were nine schools that were fully operational. We at the Maternity Center had assisted in the establishment of eight of the nine schools.

We did our first demonstration of out-of-hospital childbirth in a freestanding birth center, back in the mid-1970s. The original unit has now spawned some one hundred sixty birth centers nationwide. These centers have been established in response to the public's disenchantment with hospitals. People were having babies at home, unattended by professionals, and this wasn't safe. A birthing center is staffed by certified nurse midwives and has proven to be a safe alternative to hospital and home birth.

The original sponsors of the birthing centers feel a commitment to maintain standards in these centers, but that is proving to be a difficult task. Our problems come from physicians. On the one hand, organized obstetrics disapproves of the birthing centers; on the other hand, some of their fellows have gone into the business of birthing centers, in spades. It's lucrative and outside of regulatory hospital policies. The physicians running their own birthing centers won't listen to what we consider to be standards of safe practice. They know it all.

For example, our standards now read that there is no

place in birth centers for fetal monitors, anesthesia beyond local infiltration, or pitocin to induce or augment labor. We want to enhance natural childbirth. If the fetus is in danger, the mother should be in a hospital.

Obstetricians, in their own birthing centers, are rupturing amniotic membranes, using pitocin I.V. drips to speed up labor, and performing forceps deliveries. You name it, they're doing it. The birth center is not the place for these practices; these things should only be done in a hospital. We feel very strongly that physicians who function in birthing centers should practice midwifery—that is, the watchful waiting for the normal delivery process to occur. The birth center is not the place to use sophisticated technology.

Women want their desires recognized, and nurse midwives are prepared to help them. We take time; we place a large emphasis on how the woman feels about her pregnancy. Many women today don't trust their bodies' natural birthing responses, and we help them to be in control during those responses. We do everything possible to make childbirth an experience the woman can manage and control.

She's the star; we aren't. Midwives provide support, background information, and monitor how things are proceeding. We try to be very honest in predicting our behavior—that is, what we'll be able to do to assist the woman. We don't say, "Now let me take care of that. Just put your trust in me." We teach as much as we can about the whole experience. We trust women; we trust their bodies' natural responses.

Pregnancy provides a pretty long period of time for teaching women to become more comfortable with themselves and their bodies and what their own resources are. For me, it is a time to help the woman and her family achieve a sense of self-confidence about themselves. It's not just a matter of getting through labor—it's learning a whole childbirth and parenting role. It's helping women to see what strengths they have to parent, to use and find resources when needed. Mainly, we help them look at *themselves* as a primary resource. We are turning around the public's overdependency on health professionals.

For many years, the underprivileged were the only people nurse midwives were permitted to serve, and we did very well in serving them. Wherever nurse-midwifery services were set up, infant mortality would fall. For instance, in the sixties, nurse midwives set up a pilot project in Madera County, California. The infant mortality rate in that country was halved within the two years of the project.

The two nurse midwives were not allowed to call themselves nurse midwives; the physicians insisted they be called nurse obstetrical assistants. The California Medical Association did not permit them to continue after the two years, despite the reduction in infant mortality. As soon as the midwives left, the infant mortality rate went right back up to where it was before they came.

Another place where nurse midwives have made a profound difference is in Mississippi. A program opened there in the late sixties–early seventies. It was set up to take care of the people in Holmes County, where the mortality and morbidity rates were especially high. Bobby Kennedy had made a trip through Holmes County and suddenly things began to happen there. So a nurse-midwifery program was set up and a school was opened.

It is now closed because the physicians wouldn't tolerate it. The physician who set it up and served as a medical backup has left. That program, too, had been very successful in reducing infant mortality in Mississippi.

There are only about three thousand nurse midwives, yet organized medicine still makes a concerted effort to restrict our practice. Paradoxically, physician-extender type people, like nurse practitioners and physician assistants, continue to proliferate; they currently number somewhere around twenty thousand. Perhaps this proliferation is allowed because these people are physician-supervised. Nurse midwives have never been dominated by physicians.

* * *

I, as a nurse midwife, am in charge of the Maternity Center [MCA]. Our staff consists of five midwives and several part-time physicians. All are treated as employees, responsible to me. The physicians in the city seem unable to tolerate that MCA is hiring doctors. They'll say, "This isn't right; there has to be a physician in charge." I'll say, "Are you concerned about the clinical aspects? After all, the physicians on our payroll still have the final word in terms of clinical care."

Our medical teams review all the families every other month. The physicians have the final say as to whether the mother is high risk and should be delivered in the hospital. So there is no legitimate concern about the quality of care patients receive. Physicians, in fact, are the regulators. The battle isn't over the quality of care. The real issues are "Who's signing the checks?" and "Who's controlling the budget?"

You see, all of this is politically motivated. My doctoral dissertation analyzed barriers to innovations in health care. I used our childbearing center as a case in point. My research data show that the people in power used every trick in the book to try to close us, take our license away. They lied, saying we'd had stillbirths and maternal deaths. Receiving state Medicaid reimbursement in 1978 came after a two-and-a-half-year struggle.

Our clients are from the high-rent district now; very few, actually, are eligible for Medicaid. The ones we do get are temporarily poor—people in the arts, musicians with erratic incomes. We've been trying to take care of poor people since we got our Medicaid number. It's taken seven years to get hospital backup for our birth center on the Lower East Side. We finally got it at St. Vincent's in 1985.

I'd go to the head of hospitals with my request for backup; they'd be excited about linking with us. Then they'd go to their obstetrical attending physicians, who would squelch the idea. I have a file, yea-thick, of such encounters. One time I had a conversation with a well-known man who is in health insurance. I said to him, "Why do you think we are having so many problems? Are we threatening these physicians? Is it money? Is it power and control?"

He said, "Look, he who has the money also has the power. You can't separate the two. Power and money go together."

To be fair about it, some physicians are legitimately concerned about patients getting good care. Once we show them our track record, they come around. There are other physicians who cannot identify their sources of concern. When we were preparing to open, at a very tense advisory committee meeting, half the physicians walked off in protest. One particularly adamant physician said he could never approve the concept of a birth center. A younger man asked him, "Well, just how many safe births would you have to see in this unit before you'd approve? Five thousand? Ten thousand? How many?" The older doctor glowered at the younger man and answered, "I could never approve." The young doctor said, "Well, then, clearly safety is not the reason for your opposition, is it?" The older man didn't answer. He turned and walked away.

For a number of years, safety appeared to be the issue. The argument was, "You never know when a normal birth will become abnormal." I have to agree. That's why we practice prevention. Any suspicion whatsoever that there may be a problem with labor and we transfer the mother immediately. We don't wait. There's no second-guessing. We've had only one emergency transfer since we've been open. It was a baby boy with multiple anomalies. He wouldn't have lived even if he'd been born in the hospital.

We do not have a physician in the Childbearing Center at the time of delivery. However, every mother selects which physician and facility she'd want to be transferred to, should the need arise. We are well prepared for any emergency.

Anyone the woman chooses can come during the birth. They must see the unit before they attend the birth, however. The family goes home within twelve hours after birth; some stay only a few hours. All this flies in the face of traditional medical practices. Recently, we've opened what we call the New Family Program, which finds the mother and infant coming back for postpartum care together. Both are seen, and the mother receives class teaching during that time.

Nationwide, maternity centers come in at about forty to fifty percent of the cost of normal childbirth within a hospital. More reliance on midwifery could save the health care delivery system over a billion dollars a year. I'm not suggesting that off the top of my head. I'm quoting figures from calculated projections.

Nurse midwives are facing a new threat to their survival. Escalating malpractice rates may make it impossible for them to continue their practice. Nurse midwives always carried their own malpractice insurance whether they were employed or worked for themselves. Originally, that insurance was $29, then it went to $80, and then to $800 per year. In addition, institutional malpractice insurance rates skyrocketed, making it prohibitive for some institutions to employ nurse midwives.

Our people were still covered under the old insurance rates because they were employees. The self-employed midwives could not afford the new rates, so they no longer had malpractice insurance.

The Childbearing Center was and is covered by the joint underwriters in New York called MMIA [Medical Malpractice Insurance Association], which has been mandated to cover physicians who cannot be covered by other insurance companies. When the self-employed nurse midwives found themselves without insurance, they went to the legislature and lobbied to be included along with dentists and podiatrists who had earlier sought MMIA coverage as well.

Originally, MCA had a package deal that covered all professionals who worked in the Childbearing Center—obstetricians, pediatricians, nurse midwives, and nurses. When the self-employed nurse midwives demanded to be written into the law to receive insurance, it spotlighted all nurse midwives. The MMIA went to the Tillinghast Actuarial Consulting Service and asked for an opinion on the premiums necessary to cover midwives.

Tillinghast had very little data to draw from in terms of

nurse midwives' risk, since their experience was short in time and in numbers of women cared for. Tillinghast decided to use the record of obstetricians as a reference. Based on malpractice suits against obstetricians, they set the Childbearing Center's nurse midwives' premiums at $72,000 each per annum for one-to-three-million-dollar coverage. That's about two-and-a-half times what nurse midwives make. Even with a physician present, the actuarial consultants suggested $24,000 for nurse midwife coverage. Of course, either fee is ridiculous and far beyond what the self-employed nurse midwife can pay as well as beyond what MCA could afford. There will still be hearings because the premiums asked for were refused by the state insurance board. In the summer of 1986, the American College of Nurse Midwives was able to secure a policy with reasonable premiums [$3,500] for individual nurse midwives, but the Center is still uncertain about its coverage as a facility.

To show you how bizarre it is, MMIA doesn't care who is on the premises with the nurse midwife as long as he or she is an M.D. It can be a pathologist or dermatologist. I can't help but think that some physicians are sitting back and chuckling at our plight, hoping we'll be put out of business.

To me, the people who are most culpable in this crisis are the insurers. We met with the head of one of the largest malpractice insurance firms in the country. As soon as we walked in, he said, "I'll listen to you, but I want you to know that I'm not going to help you."

I asked this man, "Why is it that you will insure high-risk obstetricians and high-risk hospitals, but you won't insure low-risk midwives and low-risk birth centers?"

He said, "It's very simple. We can't pay more than sixty cents per premium dollar for claims. We need to know we're going to get forty cents of every premium dollar. Yes, the obstetricians are high risk, but we can predict their risk and they can afford the premiums." He didn't add, "And, lady, you can't," but I felt it was implicit. Obviously, the company's customers are the people who can afford the premiums. The more forty cents it gets, the more money the insurance company has to invest. Economically, it makes good sense. It's just not covering *our* needs.

One alternative may be self-insurance. The American College of Nurse Midwives has been looking into self-insurance. Paradoxically, the very same actuarial firm, Tillinghast, that originally projected $72,000 premiums to MMIA and created all this hassle, is now quoting desirable premiums of $3,000 to ACNM based on the same actuarial evidence. So, come on now—if someone is playing games with us, we deserve to be informed about what the rules are.

I am concerned that many nurse midwives act as though it is a sure thing that we can be self-insured. In actuality, there are still a lot of hurdles to get over, not the least of which is still the premium cost. Even if the insurance premium is reduced to $3,000 per nurse midwife, you have to remember that her salary is only about $30,000 per year at the moment.

Because the midwives secured passage of an amendment to the Risk Retention Act in the summer of '86, we can in theory be self-insured. This act allows self-insurers to sell insurance nationally without going through each state insurance department. However, such companies are very costly to capitalize and I have difficulty seeing how a small group of nurse midwives could manage such a project.

Yes, it's discouraging. Change doesn't come easily. But when I think back to the fifties, sixties, even the early seventies, and reflect on the lack of birthing choices for women then, it is apparent that we have come a long way.

Now there are a lot of choices, and among them is the whole idea of birth centers. It's caught on. We've successfully demonstrated that maternity care can be provided a lot less expensively. Our cost-effective services have gotten the attention of everybody, including the fringe benefits people in major industries, who are now writing birth centers into their health insurance packages. IBM, for example, will pay 100 percent for birth center care, whereas they have a first-day deductible for hospital birth care. Nurse midwives have been successful in getting state Medicaid reimbursement, too. We have it throughout the country.

I do regret that some nurse midwives have followed the medical model and chosen the self-employed, fee-for-service route. I know that's a natural model to follow in getting "a piece of the action," but I really regret it. In my mind, the medical model has failed to serve all of the people of this country. If we copy the fee-for-service concept, if we use physicians as our role models, we will eventually get into trouble. The medical model is focused on diagnosis and cure. You are tempted to do things because it pays and not because people need it.

I know there are also problems with health care professionals being salaried—you run into productivity problems. But, at least decisions can be made free of economic pressure on the practitioner. The employed midwife knows she will be paid, regardless. Care is her most important concern.

In addition, midwifery is an art as well as a science. Our nurse midwives are told, "If your gut tells you don't wait, then transfer the woman to the hospital." Intuition is important because health care is really an art. Practice should be based in science, but you inevitably get to that point where you cross over and your experience and intuition become very important.

Anyone concerned about nurse midwife safety needs only look at the record. If people are against nurse midwifery care, then their concern is other than safety—it's all those elements of control and so forth.

For a long time, nurse midwives have been the only ones available to the underserved. "If they are wiped off the face of this earth, who will serve the underserved?" This is the question I'll be asking in the testimony I'll be giving to the state.

19

Determination

Tessie manages a kidney transplant follow-up clinic. It's challenging work, Tessie says, because the medical episode is never over for transplant patients. The biggest battle comes after the surgery, with fighting against the body's rejection of the new kidney and the monitoring of medications.

We follow the kidney transplant recipient as soon as he is discharged from the hospital. The doctor sees the patient within a week after discharge from the kidney transplant surgery hospitalization. Thereafter, the patient sees the doctor once or twice a month.

The nurses initially follow the patient three times a week, but it really depends on the individual case. If the patient is on cyclosporin, an antirejection medicine, we must monitor him closely because the drug can be very toxic to the kidney. Since we are a regional medical center for kidney transplants, people come from all over the state and surrounding states. Our goal is to adequately teach self-care so they can safely return home.

There are some patients who initially resist seeing a nurse. They would prefer to see their doctors. They will often get mad and call the doctor, but the doctor refers them right back to us. We'll return their calls and say, "Your doctor asked us to call." Then we handle their problems. If they require further medical follow-up, we'll consult with the doctors. We want the patients to feel they can use the physician, if necessary, but what they need most, at this point, is our follow-up care.

After a while, they become confident in us and almost all of their calls come directly to us. Nurses deal with the *total* patient—the physical and psychosocial. Doctors don't usually have that kind of time. Doctors go to so many more places than we do. Because we see the patients more frequently, we are able to build a different type of relationship with the patient. For example, I recently evaluated a follow-up patient who'd had a transplant three years ago. His blood pressure was elevated, so I called him. He kept postponing his appointment with the doctor. I finally was very forceful. I told him, "You know better than that! Now get yourself in here to see the doctor." He knew I cared, so he listened. He saw the doctor the next day, and the doctor immediately admitted him to the hospital.

You need to be assertive if you are going to do your job well. One of our doctors teases me all the time. He says, "You know, if you don't get what you want from one of us, you go to someone else. You are very determined." I tell him, "You bet I am." The doctors know I care about the patient, that my observations have some merit, so they listen to me. I came into nursing after working in industry for over thirteen years. I was in charge of twenty-one people there, and I learned to be assertive in that type of job.

I feel confident in pressing my point, because it's for the patient's welfare. For example, one of our transplant patients drives a Harley-Davidson motorcycle, wears a beard, and is a real stereotype of a street-smart person. He came in, complaining of terrible abdominal pain. The doctors didn't believe him, but I did.

The doctors were saying, "He wants to be admitted just so he can get drugs." I said, "No, he lives on the street, so there's no need for him to come to the hospital to get drugs; he can get whatever he wants out there. There's something wrong with him." I continued to push until finally one doctor turned to me and said, "Just to satisfy you, I'm going to do the CAT scan you want me to do." Sure enough, they discovered a thrombosis in a vein going to the liver. They did surgery. If I hadn't persisted, he'd be dead today.

My hunch was not a gut feeling. It was a matter of being sensitive to the individual. That's my nursing contribution. In order for the doctor to do his job completely, he depends on me to pick up on subtle patient clues.

You know, when people come to the hospital, the nurse is the one they see for their care. The doctor comes in and writes an order, but if something happens to that patient during the night, it's the nurse's responsibility to know the pathophysiology, the lab results, and whatever is happening to that patient.

Nurses are the people who pick up the phone and say to the doctor, "Look, this is happening and something has to be done." Or, "I'm going to do this, that, or the other thing for this patient, and I'll get back to you and let you know what's going on."

The important thing is to listen to the patients. Yesterday I saw a patient who'd been transferred here from another clinic. I immediately observed that he became short of breath just walking from the examining table to the scale. He told me that he got dizzy every time he took a particular medication. He said he'd told the people in the other clinic about his dizziness several weeks ago, but they'd continued the medication. I told him, "This isn't right. The medication should be helping, not making things worse." I called the doctor immediately. His examination showed that the patient had pulmonary edema. He was immediately hospitalized.

Sometimes, we'll call a doctor and he'll say, "Please don't bother me anymore." When that happens to me, I'll say, "I'm not a doctor, I'm a nurse. The problem I have requires a doctor. You *must* listen." You have to remind them of their role.

Sometimes, they place so much confidence in us that they forget that certain decisions about patients are only within their domain. I will tell them, "Look, I don't want to talk to you any more than you want to talk to me! I also have important things to do. But I need your help and I need it now and you're going to give it to me now!" Consequently, we'll get on real well.

The main problem we have now, since the federal Medicare payment system Diagnostic Related Groups came in, is early discharge of patients. If a transplant patient is with an HMO not attached to our clinic, we often have communication problems. The patient may be assigned to an HMO doctor who doesn't understand the needs of kidney transplant patients.

We need to make sure that doctors out there understand the important aspects of treating transplant patients. Certain medications will cause changes in the blood picture and could cause problems to our patients. It's better for us to follow the transplant patients. Many of the physicians for HMOs recognize this and allow us to retain coverage. Otherwise, we make sure the patient thoroughly understands his care, what medications he can and cannot take. He needs to be able to protect himself. There are certain drugs that can interfere with kidney function. If the transplant patient has an infection and the local doctor prescribes certain antibiotics, the patient could experience serious problems.

Patients are leaving the hospital sooner under DRGs. I see a lot more home health care and the need for it. We work very closely with the home health care nurses that follow some of our patients. They are invaluable in caring for patients who, because of retardation, mental illness, or whatever, are unable to take their medications safely.

I started out as an associate degree nurse. I returned to school for a master's degree. I don't know . . . right now, I don't have the time. I work nine-, ten-hour days. I'm tired. I also have elderly parents whom I have to give some time to.

I would like further education, because I think it refines you. I think some of us have rough edges. Education is like sanding down a piece of wood and putting the varnish to it. When I went back to get my baccalaureate, I learned a lot of things about myself that needed to be changed. I really worked on them. There's always something else that I can work on, something that will make me a better person. Perhaps I'll be able to help someone a little bit better.

However, the patient isn't so interested in your level of education. What he wants, I think, are people who are concerned about what happens to him while he's ill.

20

No Margin, No Mission

Sister Monica, a Franciscan nun and registered nurse, has worked the last eleven years at the Guadalupe clinic, a health care facility serving the inner city's indigent populations. Most of the clinic's patients are from poor, Spanish-speaking families. The clinic, Sister Monica says, is in danger of extinction.

She speaks passionately, her casual dress reflecting nothing of her nun's habit, discarded long ago.

In the sixties, I served in the missions in Central America. The poverty we saw was horrendous. Honduras has some of the poorest people in the world. Even so, we were able to improve their health, give immunizations and food, teach hygiene, and improve their quality of life.

When I returned from the missions in the late sixties, I looked for a way to add to my nursing skills. I had learned much about physical assessment on the job, but I lacked formal training. The nurse practitioner programs were just beginning at the University of Colorado in Denver. I enrolled in the first nurse pediatric practitioner program.

This is a nurse-run, rather than physician-run, clinic. Nurses established the programs here, decided what types of health workers we needed, and went out to find people to run the clinics. We have physicians who volunteer their services, as well as some nurses. Another nurse and I are the only salaried nurses.

The advantage of this kind of clinic is that we have low administrative costs. Other clinics pay large sums of money to run their operations. This is also a limitation for us, since we didn't have the people or know-how to apply for federal monies and other supports needed to keep our clinic going. When you're taking care of patients, you don't have the time to also lobby for your interests or write grant proposals.

We offer a variety of programs here. We see healthy babies and their families. We run dental, pediatric, and obstetric clinics. We also see sick children.

We had a few other programs, but we had to cut back. HMOs have siphoned off our Medicaid patients, leaving primarily the indigent to use our clinic. You see, we refuse no one. We ask a two-dollar donation from those without Medicaid. If they cannot pay, we still see them. We cover our costs with the money we get from Medicaid and donations.

We did not apply for an HMO contract; however, as I said earlier, we didn't really have the administrative staff to do the paperwork. This means we will continue to cut our programs. By next year, we'll have to close our doors.

I am saddened over this change. Patients will be able to get care elsewhere, but they will also be deprived of a quality of care only we are able to administer.

You need to understand the culture of our people and their way of approaching care. You need to be able to communicate with them. We all speak fluent Spanish here, and we understand what kinds of things will prevent our patients from getting care.

You may tell a mother to feed her baby low-fat milk because he is getting too much whole milk and is getting overweight and anemic. She may think that, by giving him low-fat milk, she is cheating the child—sort of, "My baby deserves the finest milk"—and she'll continue with the regular milk, no matter what. Mothers who have seen children die of malnutrition believe that a fat baby is healthy. You need to build relationships with the people so they feel you have their best interests at heart, that you value them, that asking them to use low-fat milk is no put-down. I know it may sound bizarre and minor, but it is very important if you are really to improve people's health, especially for the children of the next generation.

Here at Guadalupe, we spend a lot of time teaching and building strong relationships with our people so they feel we know what we're talking about. They trust us. Our patients come back for their children's immunizations; this isn't so in some of the other clinics.

Our people also call when they're in trouble. One of our mothers, during a recent pregnancy, had a problem with her preschool child. The mother seemed to be intolerant of the child's behavior. She started to abuse the child. Because she knew we understood her, she sought out the outreach worker for help. We got her into counseling and found a temporary foster home for the child. Now the mother and child are back together and things seem to be going well. We continue to monitor the family and we can count on the mother to seek help from us. This is so because she sees us as nonjudgmental. She wouldn't seek out other people as readily.

We were able to save the lives of two children this last month, through quick thinking on the parents' and staff's part. A Spanish-speaking mother knew her child was ill—he had a temperature and a rash—and she brought him to the clinic. The doctor took one look at him and knew it was the most virulent type of meningitis—meningococcal. The doctor took the child directly to the hospital in her own car. The next day, when the nurse saw the child's sister with similar symptoms, she immediately had her admitted to the hospital. Both children were quite ill and in intensive care for several days. Of course, we never know with meningitis what aftermaths will occur.

If the mother had called the regular clinic, most likely she would have been told to give aspirin and fluids to the child. We were in direct contact and took immediate action. These are the kinds of things we do at Guadalupe.

We work with other agencies in the community. We are taking care of a child who is on a respirator in his home.

The parents are also involved in the care. Each day, for three weeks, our community outreach worker went with the child's parents to Children's Hospital, to learn how to work the machines.

You know, society still doesn't value prevention. People continue to ask, "Does good prenatal care make a difference? Do federal food supplement programs make a difference?" We know now. These programs have been markedly decreased under the current administration. What do you get? The infant mortality rate in this country is on the upswing again.

In some cities, like Chicago, infant mortality is greater than in some third world nations. What a disgrace! Besides being disgraceful, it is also a waste of human resources. We already know that poor nutrition and disease, especially in early childhood, can lead to slow learners, if not mental retardation. What lack of productivity! What treasures we are losing!

POSTSCRIPT: Guadalupe's doors are now closed due to lack of funding.

21

Nurse Anesthetists

Ross pulls bottles of beer out of the refrigerator, expertly polishes a couple of Pilsner glasses, and sits down. His muscular frame fills the captain's chair at the dining table. Just home from work, he still has on his chino slacks, an open-collared dress shirt, and docksider shoes. Within minutes, we realize that here is a man who wastes no motions, words, or time. He converses intently, breaking off only to acknowledge his daughter's arrival home from high school.

I'm an anesthetist. The difference between an anesthetist and an anesthesiologist is confusing to a lot of people. Anesthesiologists are doctors; anesthetists are nurses. An anesthesiologist spends four years in college, goes on to three years of medical school, and does a two-year residency in anesthesia. That's recently become a three-year residency. Anesthetists go through a bachelor of science in a nursing program. They go on to what amounts to a two-year residency in anesthesia.

As nurses we do things a little different from the anesthesiologists. I don't exactly know how to put it. I think that it's part of coming up through nursing, working much closer with patients on the floors than physicians do. In diploma programs, you're sometimes with patients all day.

During their training, a lot of physicians don't necessarily do that. They're more involved in classes, being in surgery, dissecting cadavers, and in physical exams of patients. The nurses I've met—and it's true of myself—have more of a personal touch than most doctors.

Without a doubt, anesthesiologists can add to the total anesthetic process for a problematic patient. They can be an asset to an anesthesia department. They have their four years of college, like I do. I went through three years of nursing school, and they went through three years of medical school.

Medical school is much more intense as far as procedure, medications, and matters like that are concerned. It's really in-depth. I mean, I had a couple of pharmacology courses, but medical school goes really in-depth. Besides that, doctors are given the clinical experience to match the use of those drugs day in and day out.

Many anesthesiologists have subspecialties, such as internal medicine or cardiology. There's no doubting that I don't have the deep background they do. Background comes in handy in that one small instance when you're in deep shit. Those extra things count.

We're safe because our association [American Association of Nurse Anesthetists] makes sure we remain current. The Recertification Council of the association requires that we take forty continuing education credits every two years, and we're recertified every two years.

There probably are not a whole lot of differences between anesthetists and anesthesiologists and what they do, other than the fact that anesthesiologists' salaries are a lot larger. As a general rule of thumb, most anesthesiologists make anywhere from three to ten times more than what most nurse anesthetists make.

Up here in Pauling, we basically do all the anesthesia that any anesthesiologist does, with the exception of a few specific neural blocks for pain control. As far as spinals and other regional blocks go, we do all of those things.

So it's a different title and a different salary, but the jobs are virtually the same. I can't tell you how recent the survey was, but according to the last figures I saw in the *Journal of Anesthesiology,* nurse anesthetists still give about fifty-four to fifty-five percent of all the anesthesia given in this country. People would be amazed if they knew this. They think the person that puts them to sleep before surgery is a physician.

I can almost guarantee that you could walk down almost any street in the United States and ask a hundred people what a nurse anesthetist is, and if you could find one or two who could even know there is such an animal, you'd be real lucky. It's amazing! In the five years I've been here, I've probably put to sleep twenty registered nurses who didn't even know there was such a thing as a nurse anesthetist. They'd call me "Doctor" and I'd say, "I'm not a doctor, I'm an R.N., just like you are." When I moved up here, my neighbors were very impressed that I was an anesthetist; if I'd told them I was an R.N. working in the hospital, I don't think that would have been the case. As a matter of fact, I'm sure it wouldn't have been the case.

An anesthetist has a great deal of respect. People call you "Mister." I have to say, "Why don't you just call me Ross?" We stand out in hospitals, and everyone knows who we are. I stand out more as an anesthetist in nursing than I do as a male in a largely feminine profession.

I've never really looked at myself as being a minority in nursing. Probably one of the reasons is that our graduating class numbered thirty-six, and fourteen of them were men. So, right from Day One, there were always a lot of male R.N.'s in our hospital.

I've never had any patients turn me down for any type of a procedure, either—as a floor nurse or an anesthetist. I guess being a male nurse is more of a rarity to other people than to me. And I don't think it is nearly as much a rarity as it was even ten years ago. On the job, being a man has never made any difference, from a patient's point of view or from another R.N.'s or a doctor's.

We have three anesthetists and an anesthesiologist at my hospital. Except for occasional calls, the anesthesiologist does not give any anesthesia; instead, he acts as a supervisor. We anesthetists do all the anesthesia. We take virtually all the call work, all the obstetrical emergencies, all the general surgery—you name it.

I really like what I do. I have a lot of autonomy. That's not true for a lot of anesthetists. Some hospitals will have an anesthesiologist who supervises a couple of anesthetists—much like we have—but it's the anesthesiologist who puts people to sleep. The anesthetists do nothing but monitor blood pressure and the vitals. Here, we totally do our own cases all the time. The anesthesiologist doesn't tell us what to do.

By law, we have to work under the supervision of an M.D. of one sort or another. Since the anesthesiologist doesn't take calls on weekends, we are considered directly under supervision, technically and legally, of the surgeon doing the operation. That surgeon may be a neurologist, a cardiac surgeon, or an orthopedic man. He almost always knows nothing about anesthesia. In a code situation or a cardiac arrest, he certainly has the same background as we do, but he probably doesn't have the expertise to help with anything directly related to anesthesia.

My job is very stressful, with long hours—frequently hideous hours, sometimes all-nighters, sometimes twenty-four hours of surgery straight through. If you screw up, I guarantee that there's a hundred percent chance of being sued. If I were making the salary an anesthesiologist makes, I think it might be more worthwhile. I mean, I'd be more willing to continue to sacrifice my body for that much money. I get a lot more than any staff nurse, but my job is only worth so much.

We anesthetists have a salary, and we also charge the hospital so much extra—a certain amount of money per hour—for the time we spend in the hospital after hours. We just turn in our hours to the payroll clerk at the hospital. We don't do any direct billing to patients.

For over ten years now, anesthetists have been fighting for direct reimbursement from patients and insurance carriers. President Reagan signed a law for direct reimbursement, but that was just for Medicare patients. A couple of states have passed laws for direct reimbursement, limited to one-year trial periods. I'm not sure if any of those states are still doing it. Here, we cannot directly bill patients. You have to be employed by a doctor, a clinic, an anesthesiologist, a hospital, or something like that. Most people think this is because the anesthesiologists have a bigger lobbying force. Our state legislature told the National Association of Anesthetists that they would just as soon not have us and the anesthesiologists compete with each other.

It's a problem of my field—you have two parties, the doctors and the nurses, who are doing the same thing. We're competing. An intensive care nurse and an internist physician certainly compete as well, to an extent, but not to the same extent as me and the anesthesiologist.

My association rationalizes the use of anesthetists to legislative health committees by saying, "One anesthesiologist costs as much as three to ten anesthetists; we're very cost effective." The association is lobbying and telling people that all the time. It's not costs or quality that keeps us from being used more; it's other issues, such as not being able to get direct reimbursement for our services.

You see, there is not a lot of public perception of nurse anesthetists. I think hospitals and doctors don't necessarily want people to know the anesthesia was given by a nurse. In general, people don't want to be put to sleep by a nurse, either. They want a doctor doing it. Frequently, the hospital is reluctant to tell people that it uses nurse anesthetists. As long as we don't bill directly, the public doesn't know what we do for them.

A lot of nurse anesthetists work for themselves, so to speak, and they contract their services to the hospital. They have their own businesses. They tell the hospital, "I'll supply your anesthesia services for X number of dollars per case or hours, or I'll work for a flat fee." They're still supervised by a physician and provide their own health insurance coverage, pensions, and malpractice insurance.

So, right now, we anesthetists are covered as employees on the hospital's insurance policy. Insurance companies will only write a limited amount for self-insurance, maybe $100,000 per case or $300,000 per year at the maximum. That's a very piddling figure. Suits for deaths, injuries, can run into the millions. Under the hospital's insurance policies, we are covered much better.

One of the reasons many hospitals have anesthesiologists

is simply for liability. The Joint Commission on Hospital Accreditation recommends that you have them. The government wants you to have them. Malpractice is taken off the surgeon's back a great deal if there is an anesthesiologist on the roster. It takes a big piece out of that lawsuit or whatever.

Still, anesthetists are as safe a bet as anesthesiologists. At a recent nationally recognized meeting, several speakers said that research shows absolutely no significant difference in the number of malpractice suits being filed against nurse anesthetists as compared to anesthesiologists. That covers morbidity and mortality nationwide.

I'm not trying to be facetious, but probably for fifty to seventy-five percent of my patient situations, my special skills were essential for the patients' recovery. Nurse anesthetists can really turn things around because of our background, or experience, and the autonomy we're allowed in our practice.

I know I can really make people feel calm when they come to surgery. Rather than being very mechanical and hooking them up to machines, grabbing orders and so on, I let the patients talk for a few minutes. I explain what I'm going to be doing. I think that comes from nursing, and maybe some of it is part of my own personality.

I've frequently seen that same type of thing in other anesthetists. It's a kind of approach. I've seen it in anesthesiologists, but I've seen it more often in anesthetists.

We used to do all of our own pre-op interviews of patients the night before the operation. Sometimes, you have to listen to a heart or the lungs. We had certain pre-op protocols we used, and we did all the post-ops. We saw everybody afterward.

Now that the anesthesiologist is at our hospital, part of his reimbursement fee is as a consult. He supervises and is there for us to consult with, if there's a problem. So he does all the pre-op visits and he does all the post-ops. We don't get out on the floors anymore. All of us really miss that. My partners and I really liked that aspect of the work, even if it was a hardship in a lot of ways. We would work all day, and then all evening we'd be doing pre-op and post-op rounds.

It made for a really long day, but it's something we would all go back to if we had a choice. We really enjoyed these rounds, plus we'd have a better rapport with the patients we were going to have in surgery the next day.

That was good for a couple of reasons. Patients would recognize you when they came into the surgery suite the next morning. Surgery is a real scary place, with lots of equipment, metal, lights, clanging and beeping sounds—you know, sophisticated equipment all over. Patients felt a lot better if they'd met you the night before, if they remembered that you'd sat and talked to them for a while in a somewhat nonclinical environment. Those things could amount to lower blood pressures when you brought them into the operating room. The individual was much more at ease. A patient misses out when the person who makes the pre-op visit is not the person who is there to put him under.

A lot of using the anesthesiologist as a consultant has to do with the government. It's set this up. It wants physicians to act more and more as direct supervisors of nurses in all areas. Eventually, the government will say there is no such thing as an anesthetist.

Today, we handle cardiac arrests on the table, severe cardiac arrhythmias, congestive heart failure, circulatory collapse, and allergic reactions. I'm particularly good at keeping anesthesia to the minimum in a procedure. All three of us are good because we can use all the various agents that are available. We really keep up. We use agents they don't even have in other hospitals.

A tremendous number of drugs and anesthetics are available if you want to use them. For years, there was "garbage anesthesia" but now, by using a combination of different things, you get a nice compounding effect. A little narcotic here, a little inhalation agent there—any one by itself would last much longer, but if you happen to be delicate enough that you can balance all these things, the patient does much better. You keep the person asleep and he won't remember. He's unconscious, relaxed, yet you can wake him in a very short time.

Waking people up quickly isn't necessarily the trick. As a matter of fact, that can be a problem. A lot of people have patients wake up during surgery. A good anesthetic means waking them up five minutes after surgery, when they're still comfortable, still stable, and don't remember. They're not having tachycardia and they're not hypertensive because of their having tremendous pain. That's a real good anesthetic. Some great anesthetics have the person asleep for ten hours, too. That's necessary in certain situations. For the majority of cases, where you want patients to come up right away, that's a real talent, a real touch.

Anesthesia, medicine, and nursing—none of those things are really a science. We call them sciences, but they're pure art . . . pure art. I don't care what anybody says. I'll argue that forever. That's particularly true with anesthesia. It's a total field of vision. I was fortunate to have trained with an anesthesiologist who was from the old school. He didn't use heart monitors or any of those kind of machines. I learned to give anesthesia by watching the patient.

Today, I can take you over there to this little Podunkville hospital here in the North Woods. We've got some of the best anesthesia equipment in the world. We have the best and the newest monitors and computers, you name it. We've got all this wonderful stuff, but it doesn't mean a damn thing because you've still got to know how much narcotic a person needs or how much inhalant or how much Pentothal or how much Valium. You've got to know that. Those machines will tell you if you're wrong, but the secret is not to be wrong!

There are some cases I've come across a half-dozen times. The last one happened during the middle of the night. A mother walked in with her baby's umbilical cord hanging out; it was a prolapsed umbilical cord. It would have been fatal to the child very quickly. The mother was in active labor, and her cervix was crushing down on that cord. I came flying in there, ran into the O.R., grabbed a mask, flipped the machine on. I had her asleep in seconds. We had the kid out in seven minutes after they called me out of bed. Another time, it took even less time—maybe five minutes. Those are neat times, because the kids would have been dead if it hadn't been for us. There's no doubt about it.

One of the things about living in a small area like this is that I have a personal relationship with these people. I know the people I care for. I've responded to I don't know how many cardiac arrests for people who are friends, people I know in the community. This is a very small town. When the patients come to, they see me and give me a big smile. They'll say, "Wow, Ross, you're here? I'm so glad." That's really nice. You walk out of the intensive care and the patient's wife gives you a big hug. Those are really nice things to have happen.

I love what I'm doing, but there are just too many other hassles, too much government intervention, malpractice—the whole thing. I can just see that in ten years I'm going to say, "That's enough." I'm sure I'll only last so long. I've thought about starting up again, as a high school teacher, making a fraction of what I make now. I want to be financially sound before I do that, though. I want my kids to be through college. I want to be fairly self-reliant, so I can afford to do it.

PART FIVE

RISKY BUSINESS

On television, hospital nurses, stethoscopes slung around their necks, charge fearlessly into crisis situations, with little concern for their personal safety. In reality, nurses are well aware of the high personal risks. Yet, for whatever reasons, nurses continue to face them.

There's Mary Ann, who jeopardizes her life to helicopter across the countryside. There's Steve, a prison nurse who wonders if the potential danger in his work will someday be realized. There's Rhea, who practiced her nursing skills in Vietnam, and whose recollections speak of a bravery not often associated with the nurse's daily life.

Working in the inner city has always been a risky undertaking but, to Marlys, the stakes have risen over the years. In the past, a nurse was given a certain amount of respect and the freedom to assist the sick and elderly without fear of harassment. Today's tough street gangs don't make such allowances.

Finally, there are the nurses who work in mental health wards. These wards are locked to protect the patient and the public, though the nurse, who is locked in with the patient, enjoys no such protection from unpredictable or hallucinating patients. Jane's story illustrates the dangers found every day by nurses on mental wards.

Working under any of these conditions is demanding

and frightening. The nurses who do it understand this and, in some cases, face the hazards of their trade. That they persevere is a powerful example of their commitment to nursing and, on a larger scale, to humanity.

22

Flight for Life

The use of the helicopter for medical rescue has come into its own in the last decade. Mary Ann, a Flight for Life nurse, is vivacious, willowy, around twenty-five years old. Her black hair is pulled back and secured at the nape of her neck with a rubber band. Her deep-blue eyes reflect the hue of her midnight-blue Gortex flight suit. Her feet are encased in huge, bulky flight boots. She looks more like a character out of Star Trek *than a nurse.*

What's my job like? To sum it up, it's hectic, sometimes scary, and often rewarding. Take the case we had one Sunday afternoon last summer. Fifty miles from here, in a small town, a young boy ran through the glass door of his kitchen. It was a freak occurrence. He severed the arteries in his armpit. The local hospital didn't have surgeons with the expertise to suture the arteries, so they called for a copter to transfer him to the medical center.

We found him in a state of shock, bleeding uncontrollably. We worked fast, infusing him with blood and transferring him to the copter. The only way I could control the bleeding was to apply manual pressure. The doc and I took turns applying pressure over the armpit and monitoring his general condition. I don't know if it was tension or what, but I pressed so hard that my arm involuntarily started to tremble. My arm was sore for days afterwards.

During the flight, the boy became "shocky." We pumped in blood, talked to him, and tried to keep him conscious. It's funny, but he was either a real stoic kid or really scared, because he hung in there and never cried.

The operating room team had been alerted and staff was waiting with the gurney when we landed. As we transferred him to the cart, he just looked at us, bleary eyed, and whispered, "Thanks, you guys." There wasn't a dry eye among us. Our flight system really worked for this kid; otherwise, he wouldn't have lived. I was exhilarated for days.

Of course, there are the times when it doesn't go well, when the patient dies in flight or later. The way I look at it, you'll never know if these people would have made it if we hadn't been there. That little boy certainly wouldn't have.

This work can be frightening. Last December, three copters went down—one in California, another in Wyoming, and one out East. No one was killed, but a pilot was seriously injured. When this happened, the whole flight network knew about it.

You can refuse to go out if the weather is bad. We usually go along with the pilot's decision. I suppose we could have a problem with the copter itself, but we all try not to think about it. Sure, we've discussed what we'd do in an emergency—say, if we had to land on water—but I usually push it from my mind. Our pilots are great, they make sure the copter is shipshape. After all, it's their life, too.

We work exceptionally well as a team, and that makes a big difference. We have distinct roles and we support each other. It's much different from what you see on the ground. As a flight nurse, my responsibility is to coordinate the team. In the air, the pilot has to fly the copter, the doctor is usually involved in technical things around the patient, so the nurse is the one to look at the whole picture. If the patient is getting shocky, the nurse needs to recognize that and suggest specific drugs. If she doesn't she can be called onto the carpet. You can't say, "Well, I knew he was shocky, but Dr. So-and-So didn't order the Levophed [medication that raises blood pressure]." It's expected that you made sure it was ordered; otherwise, you might have a malpractice problem. I used to carry a half-million dollars' worth of malpractice insurance, now I carry a million.

My relationship with the physicians is different than on the ground. Trauma specialist residents rotate through our flight service every month. As the only full-time medical person, a flight nurse is expected to show them the ropes. It's expected and appreciated. They don't resent it. In the hospital, it's a different story. Staff nurses hit a buzz saw if they try to tell a doctor what to do.

The demands on your time in this job can be a problem for women nurses with families. Right now, we work twelve-hour shifts and they're talking about going to twenty-four-hour shifts. When I have children, I don't know if I can do this kind of work, but I can't imagine ever doing anything different than emergency-type nursing.

POSTSCRIPT: Our conversation is interrupted by Mary Ann's beeper. She snatches the phone—there has been a hunting accident up north. Mary Ann moves into action. En route to the helicopter, she stops at the blood bank to grab four units of O-positive universal donor blood.

Within minutes, we reach the helipad. The physician and Mary Ann hop into the helicopter. The door closes. Quiescent, the helicopter looked like a toy, but suddenly it comes to life, as the huge blades hesitate for a split second, then rotate faster and faster. The copter lurches up, swirls into the sky, and is on its way.

23

Prison Nursing

Prison nursing is not only physically risky, but it also poses challenges to one's personal integrity. Nurses are admonished to provide unconditional care, with compassion and commitment, to all people, but most nurses never have to test the limits of their commitment. Can a nurse face the dangers of caring for murderers, rapists, child molesters, or drug dealers—day after day, year after year—without it taking a toll?

Steve has been a prison nurse for twenty years. It has not been easy. He has worked with all types of prisoners, under dangerous circumstances, and he's suffered from job burnout. Still, he projects a professional demeanor.

I began as an orderly, at the behest of the selective service! I'm a product of the sixties, and I was a conscientious objector to the Vietnam War. I'd contemplated entering the ministry after college, but I was told I'd have to do a stint in alternate service first.

I was placed at the Franklin County Medical Center for two years. During that first year, I discovered I wasn't really suited for the ministry, that my future lay in some type of health care. At the time, my fiancée was in nursing school, and I started to think I'd enjoy nursing, too, and that it would give us something in common. So I entered a two-year nursing program.

The April before graduation, my instructor tipped me off to a position at a local prison. She said, "You'd be just perfect for the job." Even now, I'm not sure what she meant by "perfect"!

I didn't know much about prison nursing. The idea intrigued me, so I went for the interview. When I got home, the look on my face gave me away. My wife said, "I guess you've found your niche." I was excited! The job fit my personality.

I tend to be someone who likes to live right on the edge. I also like to call the shots and find answers to problems, and I knew I'd be able to do that in prison nursing. My job was on the night shift. We worked independently, so far as the doctors gave us guidelines for treating specific medical conditions, and they'd OK our actions at a later time.

We have three adult prison facilities in this county—a main jail, a branch jail, and a prison farm. The main jail is a felony prison for hardened criminals—the real cruds of the world. The branch jail is for both sentenced and unsentenced people—the court dockets are so backed up that the prisoners who can't make bail may wait for several months in the branch jail. The farm is for those who are sentenced but are lightweights; they often are career criminals, your "smash and grab" types, but they're basically OK guys.

Upon entering the prison system, all prisoners are screened for medical problems. When the prisoner comes in, he meets with a triage nurse. He's asked if he has an acute medical problem, and the triage nurse decides if treatment is needed. About eighty percent of the inmates have no medical problems; we deal with the rest, the other twenty percent.

In addition to the regular staff nurses, we have a group of nurse practitioners who see patients. They augment the doctors. Many of our docs are part time, mostly senior residents from the university.

If a prisoner needs acute care, he's transferred to the university hospital and placed under guard. We can't have an intensive care unit in the prison. An ICU is like a candy factory to the prisoner. You just can't have all the equipment lying around; he'll steal it. We have a separate high-security ward for prisoners who have things like crutches, which could become lethal weapons.

If a prisoner needs follow-up care after he is initially examined, the triage nurse refers them to the staff nurses in the dispensary for therapy. Often, it's for drug therapy, to prevent seizures from drug withdrawal. Most of the people the triage nurse sees are repeaters. On any given night, we can see as many as fifteen new people, in addition to our regulars. And emergencies can always occur.

At five A.M. on a typical day the prisoners are counted. The deputies take the booking picture of the prisoner and see if it matches up to the inmate in the cell. After the count, we start the glucometer testing of the diabetics, draw up their insulin. We don't use the inmates' own supply of insulin, because it frequently is laced with another drug. I can remember one fellow who had a vial that actually looked muddy. We sent it out for analysis and found a high concentration of heroin.

After that, we pass the tranquilizers to the wackos. We check to see that people don't hoard their pills. Though we have licensed practical nurses and guards helping us out, we still don't have enough help to do all the checking. Tranquilizers are given in liquid form; otherwise, the inmates might hoard them to overdose on a later date.

During the early morning, we have a lot of drop-in "emergencies"—people who say they don't feel well or have the sniffles, stuff like that. Most of the time, these are not real emergencies, but the deputy will not screen them for us. It gets frustrating when you're trying to deal with a real emergency, like an asthmatic attack, when you get a guy who wants attention for a stuffed nose.

We have what we call "snivel sheets." Every inmate has the opportunity twice daily to come to sick call. It's sort of a social time for a lot of these guys. If they get away with it, they'll fake some symptom just to get to sick call.

As you can imagine, with all the chemical abuse, we have a lot of psychiatric problems. We have a psychiatric unit, equipped with a complete in-house psychiatric team. As harsh as it sounds, the goal is not so much to completely cure or rehabilitate those guys as it is to make them sociable enough to be integrated back into prison life.

Some people would say, "Aren't you gonna get them well enough to walk on the streets?" I look at them and say. "Sorry, they aren't going on the streets." With the medical services we have, we are lucky if we get them well enough to participate in prison living and court hearings. You know, they didn't get to us just because they're wackos; they've committed a crime—often a heinous crime.

Almost ninety percent of our prisoners have some type of addiction. They really don't want to kick their drug and alcohol dependency. In jail, they're forced to withdraw because they can't get the stuff. Medically speaking, we take what steps are necessary to get them through it. For the most part, coming off drugs isn't that bad. With very rare exceptions, heroin addiction is easier to kick than cigarettes. Physical withdrawal is like a very bad case of a seventy-two-hour flu, and to my knowledge there has never been a death from heroin withdrawal. Once they get over the hump, only the intense cravings and some sleep disturbances go on for several weeks.

In cocaine addiction, there are no real physical withdrawal symptoms, so we ignore it completely. With alcohol, however, you have a whole different story. It is a killer! The d.t.'s are terrible. We use Serax, a drug which has a calming effect. We have A.A. meetings and social workers to make referrals for follow-up treatment after discharge. Problem is, most of the lightweights are in jail for such a short time that none of this is effective.

Most of the prisoners don't recognize their alcoholism and drug addiction as a problem. They see their lifestyles as being every bit as legitimate as yours or mine. That's the one thing that surprises most of the new nurses. They come in here thinking, "We'll help those poor souls kick their habits and have a better life." On the whole, criminals don't think their lives on the outside are that awful.

Unfortunately, during the sixties and seventies, we accepted all the crud fed to us by the media and psychologists —ideas about free spirits and the notion of finding oneself.

Society justified deviance—"These people weren't loved." Or, "They were just potty-trained too late."

What it really comes down to is, at some time in their lives, they made a free choice not to live by the rules, and now they're reaping the "rewards" of their choice.

Attempted suicides are not unusual here. Most suicides are staged, and they occur around ten at night, or in the early morning. I've run into a heck of a lot of those. The successful suicides are usually accidents. The inmates do it to get your attention. It's a gesture. Some guys are successful and some are not. They can always get a sharp instrument, or they can make one. These are exceedingly clever people. They have nothing else to do but think up ways to do themselves in, if that's their desire.

One of the most dramatic suicides I can recall happened when the fellow was in protective custody for attempting to hang himself. He was a multiple child molester, and he had made several attempts to kill himself before.

It was during the big count at five A.M. The deputy threw the lights on, went down to the inmate's cell, and found him in a sea of blood. When I say "sea," I mean the cell floor was completely covered. He'd exsanguinated. The deputy immediately gave the signal for "man down."

When "man down" happens, you never know what you are getting into. It might be a knifing, a suicide, or a prison riot. You get there quickly, with no questions asked. I tore down to the cell, saw the mess, and asked, "Are the paramedics rolling?" They said, "No." I said, "Well, you sure as hell better get them rolling now, buddy."

I couldn't believe that the guy still had a faint pulse. I could barely make out if he was breathing. I took a quick look over the whole body to see if I could find the wound. At first, it was difficult; his whole body was caked with blood. I finally located the wound in the brachial area of his arm. He'd tried to get the artery but he'd cut the vein instead. So instead of blood shooting out like a garden hose, it trickled. This cat really meant business; he had leaned over the toilet and pumped his arm, expelling blood until he passed out cold. The remainder of his blood slowly trickled onto the floor of the cell. We got him to the hospital emergency room, but they lost him there. It was just too late.

These prisoners are people who have no compunction about killing another human being. The heavies are escorted by a guard when they come for health care. Some people feel that the guard's presence violates the prisoner's privacy. To heck with privacy! My safety and my life are more important than any prisoner's privacy.

I've had many skirmishes that scared the daylights out of me. Some of these were with prisoners who were actually psychotic. I recall one mealtime when I was passing medications alongside the trusty with the meal tray. This particular inmate grabbed the trusty and threw him clear across the cell. The deputy came running. The prisoner was mammoth in size and had the strength of Goliath. He knocked the deputy down with one swift blow. The deputy, stunned momentarily, recovered and pushed the prowler signal. When the prowler signal is sounded, every available person comes running. It sounds like a herd of buffalo but, believe me, you're glad to hear that racket. Meanwhile, the prisoner had turned on me. I was smaller than he, but I was able to get a choke-hold on him. You know, if you press on both carotid arteries you can knock a person out. I didn't have a tight enough hold to knock him out, but it was enough to make him dizzy. It took about fifteen seconds for deputies to restrain him, but it seemed like an hour.

On another occasion, the inmate had just been released from isolation. Some smart guy on the psych team thought the prisoner needed "socialization." The prisoner pounced on a deputy, broke his nose, and knocked him out. Next, this fellow spies one of the nurses, a very sweet Filipino gal who was barely five feet tall. He lunged for her. I was coming down the hall and caught the scene. I immediately pounced on the guy and did the choke hold, which was tight enough this time to knock the guy out. This time, there was no prowler button, and the other nurse yelled for help. Meanwhile, the deputy was bleeding like a stuck pig. There was blood all over the place, all over me.

How do I feel about giving care to these people? Any of us may have a revulsion toward crime, but we still provide the care. Most of the time, we don't even know why the fellow is in prison. We need to know only if it bears on his health history—like drug addiction, for instance. Sure, nurses and prisoners have conflicts, but they usually stem from personality conflicts.

Working in prison nursing has taught me that I don't have the power to reform anyone. I recognize that the majority of these people do not want to reform; they don't see any problem with their lifestyles. In fact, they laugh at the straight life.

I was recently transferred from the branch to the prison farm. I was getting burned out. I hadn't realized it until an article I'd written about how I practiced as a prison nurse was published in the *American Journal of Nursing.* Several of my friends came to me and said, "This isn't you, Steve; You don't practice this compassionately now." I had to admit they were right.

I was startled when I came to the realization that the person in the article was no longer me. A lot had happened in the five years between the time I'd written the article and when it was finally published. I had to take another look at myself. Who was I? Where was I going? I was becoming hardened. I no longer liked myself.

My transfer to the farm has been a lifesaver. I'm the only nurse for eleven hundred prisoners at night. The people I care for are not hardened or dangerous criminals. You can talk to them, one human being to another. You don't feel that your life is constantly in danger.

For the few prisoners who do question their existence, we can provide support in their quest for a more meaningful life. It doesn't happen often; in fact, it's rare. It's only happened twice in my time. To miss this miraculous feat, whether through indifference or contempt, is to miss the greatest reward of one's career.

In my religious faith, we look at troubles, problems, and travails as tests that must be passed before we can move on.

It is through these tests that we learn. If we don't pass the test, it will be given again and again until we do pass. We also believe that God never tests us beyond our capacity. Sometimes—often, in fact—the test requires that we dig down deep within ourselves, as well as reach out to our fellow man and to God. That is what both of these men did, and that is why they succeeded. I had little to do with their success. I was just the fortunate observer.

24

Vietnam and Beyond

Rhea is tall and statuesque. Her hair, graying at the temples, is fashioned in a closely cropped Afro. She holds a master's degree in nursing.

I need to go back twenty-plus years to tell you how I got to Vietnam. I was enrolled in a baccalaureate nursing program at Tuskegee. I come from a family of ten, so there wasn't much money for school. My counselor suggested that working during nursing school would be difficult, given the rigors of the program, and she suggested that I consider joining the Army Student Nurse Corps. The Army would finance my education and give me a small amount to live on.

Serving time in the Army was not a thought I relished. I *dreaded* the idea. I was part of the sixties crowd; in fact, my dean thought I was rather radical. I guess I had a free spirit! I wanted to be a lot freer than the Army would allow, but I had no feasible alternative, so I joined. After graduation, to pay back my commitment, I was required to enter the military on a full-time basis.

After three months as an Army staff nurse, I was placed in a head nurse position. I didn't get this position because of my experience. It was due to my education; there were few degreed nurses available.

This was the mid-sixties. The war in the Far East was

building up. It was no longer feasible to send the wounded back to the States, so plans were made to take care of the wounded near the site of battle. I was assigned to a hospital in Japan that had been used during World War II and was in dire need of renovation. In fifty days, our team converted this seventy-five-bed hospital into a five-hundred-bed facility. Needless to say, there was marked expansion and crowding.

After six months in Japan, I had a chance to come back to the States if I so chose, but I was curious about what was actually going on at the front. I guess I wanted to see how I could help the critically wounded. So I volunteered for Vietnam.

When I got to 'Nam, I was made a head nurse over five wards—Malaria, GU, Neuro, Ortho, and General Surgery. It was, as we like to say, quite an experience. We worked fourteen to sixteen hours a day. I stayed there for ten months and then came back to the States.

At this point, her voice lowers, as if she is having some difficulty with the memories of her experiences. For now, she doesn't wish to volunteer information about what transpired in her ten months at the front. Instead, she talks of her return to the States:

In the States, I was able to take advantage of the "Token Black Era." My promotions were rapid: I got every assignment I asked for. I was selected for what is called a "charm school" course, which was a course for people who will stay in the military and who have potential for advancement. The course involved study of the computer sciences as well as business and management skills. From there, I went to Valley Forge and taught medical corpsmen. The war in Vietnam was still going on, and there was a dire need for medics. Since physicians were not brought to the front lines, the Army needed the medics to take care of the wounded. My job was to train the medics to function as physicians. As soon as the medic graduated, he was shipped to Vietnam.

I taught this program for two years. I was getting bored, and I was looking for another assignment. My brother was in the military, and he was scheduled for Vietnam. As you may know, the military doesn't send two people from the same family into a combat area during the same time, and since my brother had small children, I volunteered to return to Vietnam in his place.

The first time I was there, I was stationed in a hospital about two hundred fifty miles from Saigon, a place called Qui Nhon. It was like what you've seen on *M*A*S*H.* You learned to make do with very little. We had more patients than equipment. You also learned to train nonprofessionals, such as corpsmen, on the spot. We nurses placed catheters into main arteries and did a variety of other intrusive procedures—many of the things that nurses stateside are not allowed to do. Necessity brought out the best in people, and you quickly learned to be adept in areas you never dreamed you had skill in.

We didn't have many physicians—or nurses, for that matter. We learned to make quick assessments and institute procedures, with or without physician orders. Otherwise, it was the boys' lives. Most of the time, I had two nurses and five units, with thirty-three beds each.

At night, one nurse actually covered all the units. If a patient went bad, the nurse could be tied up and you had to depend on the corpsmen. The nurses often assumed physician duties and the corpsmen assumed the nurses' duties. You had to get along with each other because you depended upon each other, and because you worked long hours in close proximity. Even so, racial prejudice continued. I knew black corpsmen who went to the NCO and were beaten by the whites there.

Women were few and far between, and nurses were really respected. You got to know those guys; you were like a mother, or a big sister, to them. They'd tell you about their experiences in the fields, the horrors and their nightmares. It was important that what you did as a nurse was good. There was no way you let the guys down.

I remember the first time I flew into Saigon. It was monsoon weather, and we had to circle before landing. I thought, "God, this is it!" It was scary getting on and off planes. The Vietnamese would bomb the airports and planes at landing or takeoff. Several of our people survived the battles, only to be killed getting on a plane for the States.

The hospital in Qui Nhon was a scary place. In order to get to the hospital from our quarters, we needed to go through a Vietnamese village. That was frightening because you never knew who was lurking there, ready to kill you. The enemy had no respect for the hospital or the wounded. The Vietnamese would sneak into the hospital and plant plastic bombs in the latrine. Or we'd get sniper fire.

Another danger was the location of the hospital. They were often built close to an airstrip or ammo dump. I guess the rationale was that the enemy wouldn't bomb those areas because of the hospitals. Heck, they didn't care. They were always bombing airstrips and ammo dumps.

Qui Nhon was like a fortress. On one side were mountains infested by Vietnamese; on the other side was the harbor to the sea. The warships were moved there. No place was safe. There was always a chance for attack from the mountains, sea, or air.

During my second experience in Vietnam, we had nurses who weren't able to withstand the rigors of combat. A few had nervous breakdowns. It wasn't easy seeing those fellows come in with their pelvises shot to pieces or their guts spilling out or their heads shot off and their brains oozing out.

The working conditions were also rough. The quarters were what one might consider slum conditions. I recall a nurse recruit who had been with us a little over a week. She was into redecorating her room. For some reason, the previous occupant had placed burlap over one wall. As the recruit proceeded to remove the burlap, thousands of roaches started swarming all over the place. She freaked out—went completely berserk—so she had to be shipped out.

A chief nurse had a complete psychotic break. Sure, she had problems already, but the environment triggered her final break. Fortunately, those situations were rare. We really *are* a pretty resilient people and are able to tolerate much more than anyone would believe the human psyche can take.

None of us were prepared for what we saw or had to do, but we did it. In that regard, I'm not concerned about our ability to exist. What I am concerned about is the type of war that will be fought in the future. It's predicted that the next war will not be like any other fought in the history of mankind. It will be a biological, chemical war. The first seventy-two hours will tell the story—if we don't survive that length of time, all will be over. Our people train, with limited equipment, on the average of once a year; the Russians train often, with complete equipment.

It's the same in health care as in the military. I have continued in the reserve, training medics to be combat ready. From my observations in the military hospitals, I would say that the health care drastically changed between 1965 and now. Frankly, I would not recommend a military hospital today. Lots of money is being used for high administrative costs, to the detriment of personnel budgets, appropriate training, and supervision.

Would I go back again? I guess that question is rhetorical. If it's a chemical war, who wants to exist anyway? I hope to God I never need to find out.

25

Working in the Inner City

Marlys is a city public health nurse in her mid-thirties. She works our conversation into her busy day's caseload. As we sit down, she shows us her public health badge, prominently displayed on her sturdy black bag.

In years gone by, she tells us, an unwritten street code allowed nurses wearing the badge to pass unharmed through the tougher neighborhoods. Today's street gangs jeer at this unwritten code.

My district covers four long by six short city blocks. I function as a school nurse for approximately twelve hundred children attending the district's two schools. The elementary school includes two learning disability classes, two classes for emotionally disturbed, and two preschool classes. Many of these children are not even potty-trained when they come to the school.

The six hundred students at the middle school attend sixth to eighth grade and, on any given day, I will get a one-and-a-half-page, single-spaced printout of the truants. Last year, during a period between Christmas and January first, we diagnosed twelve new pregnancies from that school. These are all high-risk kids without any of the bases covered in prenatal care except for my one-to-one teaching.

Each district nurse runs two clinics a week, where we do health-risk screening, physical assessments, lifestyle counseling. During the remainder of my time, I do home visits to the families in my area. I teach geriatrics, diet, meds, treatments, and mental health, and I make referrals to other health professionals. It's hard to draw a clear line between social work and some of the things we nurses do.

I get involved in a lot of child and woman abuse and child neglect situations. Of ten new mothers in the district, eight will have high-risk infants or will have problem deliveries—a reflection of the drug and alcohol abuse. Lots of mothers I see have been on alcohol or drugs throughout their entire pregnancies.

In the last two years, the district has changed drastically. Drug use has doubled; the district has become unsafe. Funding for programs has been cut back. There is much more crime, much more despair. Truancy is up. Even if the kids go to school, it's not unusual to see them, as young as ten years old, dealing drugs on the way to school. If a child grows up halfway decent, he is growing up despite his home situation.

The dangers in our district are very real. The neighborhood isn't the same as it was in the sixties. People used to respect the Public Health uniform, but not anymore. In order to survive, we need to become much more streetwise. You need to know your district like the back of your hand. You have to know every person as well as which places are safe to go into and which are not. We informally share that kind of information with each other.

One young nurse was not streetwise and she finally had to transfer out. She would wear frilly blouses on the job. A man put his hand on her knee through the car window while she was waiting for a traffic light. She didn't anticipate that. We are taught to avoid situations that are not correct.

I let my guard down last spring. A youth gang came after me. I saw them on the street, in the usual place, before I went in to see a client. When I came out, they had moved. I should have realized then that something was up. By the time I got to my car, the gang was closing in on me. Foolishly, my one thought was to get into the car. I should have gone back to the house and called the police.

I had my hand on the car door when this big guy put his hand over mine. My other hand was on my bag. He looked at me, at the mace in my bag, and again at me. He hesitated, trying to decide if I'd use it. My client was on the porch, and there were a couple of others yelling at the gang members from their windows. Neighborhood people will look after you if they like you. Color doesn't make a difference. The big guy backed off. I got in the car and drove out of there. The gang realized that there were too many witnesses. They threw a board at the car as I drove off.

I reported it to the police and took the rest of the day off. I couldn't work. It was a couple of weeks before I got up the nerve to go into that section alone. For weeks, I took a city escort with me. One day, the city actually sent a dog-catcher with me as an escort.

Even though it can be dangerous, I love public health nursing. It's a different kind of nursing. The clients are in control. When you're in their home, you're their guest. The clients don't have to let you in if they don't want to. I've scheduled appointments with clients who are away from their homes when I arrive. After a year of this, they'll suddenly let me in. They'll say. "If you care enough to keep coming back all the time, I should do what you want."

We have the worst area in the city, and we're told that no visit is more important than our own safety. The police say we should not ever be out there alone. Our union requested a formal list of names and addresses in the district where you might have trouble—places to be visited only with police. The agency assigns two nurses when necessary, but I don't know how much longer that will last, the way the money is drying up. I wonder what will happen if we no longer can go into the homes when people need us.

26

Danger Zone

We ring the bell at the Mental Health Unit. Through a small window in the door, we can see Jane striding toward us. Reaching into her pocket, she pulls out a set of keys secured by a cord around her waist. She unlocks the door and escorts us past a row of single-patient rooms. She unlocks the staff office door at the end of the corridor and motions for us to enter. The automatic door lock clicks shut. In the security of this small office, we are shut out from the world of the mentally ill.

My mother took her own life a few years ago and I guess I was drawn to mental health nursing as a way to work out some of my own emotional responses to her tragic death. It's helped. I've learned a lot about myself, and I understand other people better.

This is a state institution, and it has all the problems of a bureaucracy. I don't know what it is about a state mental hospital, but a lot of weirdos work here. Some of the staff are as sick as the patients. One of the nurses I worked with before coming to this unit was like that. She'd run around the unit, trying to do everything and getting nothing done. She and I had some real conflicts over patient routines and patient control measures.

Patients know when staff are having conflict. Consequently, there was a lot of acting up by patients on that unit

—yelling, resisting staff directives—things like that. This tense atmosphere created more agitated patients, so more seclusion times and restraints were necessary. On one particular day, the nurses were exchanging change-of-shift reports. We heard someone shouting. I tore out to investigate.

Jake, a patient about six feet tall and weighing about a hundred seventy-five pounds, was obviously hallucinating. His eyes lit on me. "You're the one they told me to get!" he shouted. I didn't bother to find out who "they" were. My only thought was to get the hell out of there.

I wasn't fast enough. He came at me with all his might and slammed me against the counter of the nurses' station. It's a four-foot-high counter that divides the hall like a soda fountain counter.

Jake knocked me dizzy. He came at such a fast pace that, after he hit me, he sort of pole-vaulted over the counter and landed flat on the floor inside the station.

Lorna, the nurse standing inside the station, lifted a chair, ready to hit him if he continued his violence. Well, Jake just got to his feet, looked around in sort of a daze, and sauntered away.

It was terrifying for everyone. You know the superhuman strength of mental patients when they get out of control. Everyone could see what was coming, but there was no stopping it. I was practically knocked out. At first, they thought I had broken ribs. Fortunately, there were only contusions. I was sore for weeks. I felt like my body had been thrown off its axis. Even now, after nine months, my feet and ankles still hurt a lot.

I was lucky. The worst assault happened a few months ago. A patient went berserk and attacked a nurse with a fork. He got her in the neck and just missed her carotid artery. She was off work for several weeks. Then, just last month, a nurse on another unit was sexually assaulted. The patient grabbed her and started ripping off her clothes. She could have been raped.

I'm no longer on that unit. I'm now on a new teaching unit, which has a real team spirit. It's much better staffed, and I expect to see some good coming out of my work.

Besides staffing problems, the other thing that bothers me about working here are the present mental health laws. Currently, unless people are dangerous to themselves or others, patients cannot be committed without their consent. The law was enacted to protect people from inappropriate incarceration, but the problem is that too many mentally ill people lose touch with reality and may do things such as going outside in winter with just a dress on, or neglect to eat or take their medications.

Recently, one of our patients—who should have been committed—was found dead. We knew she had problems. She had a seizure disorder along with her mental illness. She frequently would go off her medications. They found her dead outside her house. She'd had a seizure.

That's why I'm down now. We all felt so bad about her death. Maybe we should have pushed more for her commitment, so she could have received proper care. I keep hoping that next time we will be more successful with patients like her. Maybe next time we can save a life.

PART SIX

EXPLORING NEW HORIZONS

Within the citadels of medical practices, nurses who are not treated as trained professionals either change their work settings, shape nontraditional roles, or opt out of nursing entirely. Those who are risk takers may start their own business or explore new horizons in health promotion, rehabilitation, or wellness. These nurses structure their new territory according to their uniqueness as a person, their accumulated nursing knowledge, and their highly transferrable managerial skills.

Are nurses who no longer directly concern themselves with clinical care still considered nurses? Dyed-in-the-wool nurses, wed to their clinical practices with patients, would say that they should not be. But science—including the science of nursing—is not just a collection of facts and formulas. Science integrates the phenomena of human experiences within the practitioners' system of beliefs. Scientific knowledge becomes useful as a discipline's practitioners design techniques appropriate to their belief system. Is an engineer still an engineer after forsaking the drafting board to head a company? How well can anyone be divorced from a discipline once its scientific techniques and beliefs have been acquired?

In this section, we hear from nurses who have pursued other avenues outside the profession, combining what they're learned from nursing with innovative directions in health care. Each voice represents an element of nursing not often associated with the profession in the public eye, yet each voice is undeniably a part of nursing, in the present and the future.

27

Entrepreneur

We are sitting on the screened-in porch of Margaret's home. While we enjoy an afternoon snack, Margaret enthusiastically details the building of her nurse business for us.

Becoming an entrepreneur happened by accident. I have over twenty years in hospital nursing; my last job was as a director of patient care services. The hospital changed administrators and everything changed for me. It was evident that there was a need for a changing of the guard. My departure was not only inevitable but necessary.

It was not easy to leave secure surroundings with no definite road map to another job. Anxiety and fear were my constant companions for many months. Where did I belong? What did I want to do? Being plagued by a lack of self-confidence, coupled with heavy doses of self-pity made decision making a painful process. However, the need to survive financially left me no choice but to go out to find work.

I have a master's degree in business administration, as well as many years of administrative experience. Nurses were starting businesses around the country, so I decided to give it a try.

At first, my idea was to have a nurse group practice. Nurses would run the business. But the market wasn't right for selling nurses' individual skills. You can have great ideas, but if the market isn't right, your ideas won't fly. The entrepreneur is a person who takes something and makes something out of it. It is looking to see what is needed and developing the idea—like Federal Express or Pizza Hut. If you're going to be an entrepreneur, you've got to be an opportunist. You need to identify the market needs and sell your services to meet those needs. It was the late seventies when I started out, and the nursing shortage was acute. Hospitals desperately needed nurses. I capitalized on that need and started a nurse-staffing business.

My resources were limited. I had about two thousand dollars in the bank. In addition, my elderly mother lived with me and was dependent on me. I knew the Small Business Administration gave loans, particularly to women starting businesses. I approached the Small Business Administration and was given a $20,000 loan.

The first thing I did was contact an advertising agency that helped to develop the business name, logo, stationery, and business cards. Then I set up a small office in my home. Since it was necessary for me to stay close to home, and because I had established contacts here, I decided my market would be in the country surrounding my residence.

I started out by providing nurses for nursing homes. Later, I moved into critical care. Currently, we have about eighty nurses working full and part time.

Our type of agency is very viable in today's health care market. It's more feasible for hospitals to cut core staffs and fill in with temporary staff to meet short-term increases in census. Another reason we're viable is the current shortage of intensive care nurses. In 1984, few new grads were hired. The hospitals decided not to accommodate for attrition, so they had no replacements. Even though the hospital census had fallen steadily since DRGs, hospitalized patients are, on the whole, much sicker than before. Many require intensive care nursing. Since few nurses were hired in 1984, we are now seeing an acute shortage of nurses prepared to work in intensive care. Consequently, in some cases, we provide as much as seventy-five percent of our clients' intensive care nursing staff.

What has worked very well for us is private duty. We

take care of very complex cases in the home, such as patients on respirators. Right now, we're providing twenty-four-hour-a-day care to a lady who wishes to die at home. She's receiving artificial feedings through her veins, as well as several other complex therapies.

Our contracts provide her nurses who put in a lot of hours and can make a continuous commitment to these people. We feel sure about our nurses, and our reputation is good. At first, we did an extensive profile on a nurse and gave it to the institution in which she worked. The people in the institutions liked it so much that they used the profile information to recruit the nurses. We stopped that! After all, business is business!

Many of our people have at least a baccalaureate degree. We particularly like the nurse who is back in school, working on an advanced degree. Somehow, they seem to be more motivated. In general, we attract a nurse who is self-motivated and not afraid to be on her own in new situations.

Since the majority of our business is in critical care, we maintain a vigorous screening process, including a skills assessment checklist and a written test. We prefer nurses who are certified in critical care.

The institutions like dealing with us. It's cost effective—they have the potential for saving the wages of a staffer as well as the costs of orientation, turnover, and fringe benefits.

The nurses like working through agencies. They pocket more cash this way. If they are on a hospital payroll, they participate in the regular and usually mandatory fringe benefits program. Some nurses might want the fringes; my group doesn't. Some are married and derive benefits from their husbands' employers; others are going to school and are willing to forfeit the benefits in lieu of the additional cash.

Some people argue that you don't have commitment from the nurse in this type of staffing arrangement. That's nonsense. Our staff is less bound by the institutional structure and can be more committed to the patient. Actually, this system is not new. Years ago, nurses were free agents, hired by the patient on a case basis. In fact, this is the private duty nurse concept.

Staffing hospitals is a horrendous job. Hospitals find they need a two-tiered system: one that provides their own internal staffing, and a second that uses freelancers from agencies such as ours. The problem is, there are prejudices toward the outside agency concept. People see agency nurses as "temporaries." The connotation of a temporary is like the idea of an "appliance nurse"—the nurse who is working to buy the refrigerator, the washing machine, and so on. We think of our nurses as freelancers. They go from job to job at their own will. By the same token, you expect the freelancer to be a professional who is as committed as the regular staff.

Another problem is professional jealousy. Some staff nurses resent the freelance nurse because the freelancer can call the shots in terms of the schedules they'll work. That's one reason why some hospitals won't allow a nurse who was previously employed by them to return to work as a freelancer. It's not because they are incompetent, but that it may cause dissension among the staff.

You learn the value of the dollar when you run a business. I didn't make my own salary for the first three years; I had the cost of running the business and paying the nurses. I've been in this for a little over six years. It wasn't easy to hang in, but when I considered the alternative of working in the hospital system, I decided the sacrifice was worth it.

It's lonely being in business for yourself. I structured a support system by contacting other businesswomen. I contacted a successful businesswoman who runs a professional support group. I also consulted a Chicago nurse who has her own critical care nurse staffing business. She helped me to develop the screening tests for the critical care nurses we hire. I can't stress how important it is to reach out for help. You do have doubts at times. Starting my own business was very frightening, especially at my age. After all, how many times can I start over?

If you're going to be successful in your own business, you need to have a mindset that says, "I will continue to grow." You don't set a cutoff for that growth. That is, you can't say.

"I'll only grow until I'm making $30,000 per year." You need to think that you'll continue to grow, at whatever cost.

Success perpetuates more activity. Once I got going, I was stimulated to think about ways to expand. I now have two offices and I'm exploring the idea of setting up an agency in another part of the state. Once you're successful, you believe in yourself. Things start to happen—you *make* them happen.

It's fascinating and challenging. I'd like to expand into other areas besides nursing. For example, right now, down by our lakefront, there is a real need for some gourmet-type picnic baskets. The area is developing and a business could do well there. I'm thinking about starting one. My problem is that I'm overcommitted now. I need to bring in another manager if I'm going to expand.

I'm not alone in believing nurses should be entrepreneurs. This type of business is growing around the country. They, like I, believe nurses have a right and responsibility to benefit from their contributions to organizations. We can also deliver better patient care if we are calling the shots.

I'm a realist. Everyone talks about working in collaborative relationships with physicians, but I've failed to see it. Nurses have bought into their own rhetoric. Just think of the wonderful things that could happen in health care if nurses could do what they've been educated to do without the undue constraints they currently face in toady's health care system.

Nurses are getting tired of being restricted. That's why I believe many smart nurses are leaving nursing. They are women, like me, who have the wherewithal to have independent success.

A lot of nursing's problems are our own. As a group, we are not risk takers. That comes partly from our work experience. You cannot risk when you are caring for patients, and that carries over into other areas of our lives. Instead of taking a stand and demanding to exercise an autonomous role, we create artificial structures to fool ourselves. We go through all kinds of game playing to make ourselves believe we're really in charge.

Our head nurses are no longer head nurses—they're patient care coordinators. What does *that* mean? Has the system changed so she can coordinate care? No. For the rest of the hospital, it still means her getting the patient down to X-ray to fit in with the X-ray department's schedule, not the patient's nursing needs.

One problem is we don't value ourselves. Recently, I was talking with a nurse practitioner who works with a physician. I said to her, "Don't you think your services are worth at least forty thousand dollars a year? After all, you're an important adjunct to his practice." She acknowledged that she was good enough to take the physician's place in many instances, but she was unwilling to fight for a fair share of the income.

It saddens me when I talk to people like this. I wish they would recognize the importance of their contributions to the health care system.

28

Marketing Health Care

Ryan's office in the Jefferson County Mental Health Complex boasts all the appointments normally associated with a thriving medical business. The only clue to his former ties to nursing is the inscription "Nurse of the Year" on his coffee mug.

Were opportunities greater for me because I was male? Not really. The only perk I ever had for being male was that I was admitted to the university nursing program in three days. That was a first—they were anxious to fill their minority slots.

My wife was a nurse, so I knew all about nursing—or I *thought* I did. It seemed to be a steady way to make a living and a good way to pay something back to society. What really attracted me were the many avenues open to nurses, as compared to other fields.

My first semester in school, I lived on my savings, but then I had to look for some source of income. I was fortunate to land a hospital position helping the nurses weigh patients before breakfast. I did that for a little over a year. Early morning is a quiet time in the hospital. I got to talk to a lot of people. I learned quite a lot about the organization and the people who work there.

I wanted to learn more, so I approached the clinical director of the open heart unit and asked if they had a job for me. I thought this would add to my student nurse experience. The director decided that I could be trained to operate a couple of machines in the unit. I worked weekends and holidays until I finished school. My teachers might be surprised by my saying so, but I think I learned as much during those work experiences as I did from my formal education. In school, we didn't spend enough time with patients to become proficient in an area. In fairness, I realize that it probably isn't possible in the allotted time. If you were to become proficient in all areas of nursing, you'd need to lengthen the program from four to six years.

After graduation, I completed a nurse internship in critical care. After a while, I decided that I needed to get away from the intense environment of critical care. Since psychiatry was the only area I didn't have experience in, I decided to try mental health nursing. The typical psych nurse doesn't know or feel comfortable with the physical care of patients, so they were glad to have someone like me.

I noticed that patients had a real lack of understanding of their medications and how to take them, as well as of their side effects. I saw a real need to teach patients these things. I couldn't believe the resistance I received from the psych nurses. They only believed in nursing the patients' psyche. Well, I believed in that, too, but if you believe in taking care of the whole person, you need to deal with his physical needs as well. If a patient on "mood elevators" doesn't understand the need to maintain his medication blood levels, or if he doesn't know the side effects of the drugs, it can be pretty serious.

In retrospect, I think the psych nurses didn't want to see a new person come in and rock the boat. The nursing profession, whether you are front line or management, is extremely stressful. Nurses get caught in the middle all the time—between doctor and the patient and family. You are paid to take care of the patient, but everything else gets in the way. So when somebody new like me comes in with a new idea, staff just can't adapt. I stuck around there for a year and a half, but I was a single person and I couldn't buck the system. I decided that if I were the manager, I wouldn't get so much resistance. The staff would need to do what I directed—I'm sure you've heard that pipe dream before!

I took a job as a second-shift supervisor in a nursing home. I was divorced by then, and working that shift made it easier for me to see my children. Four years ago, the nursing home had been bought out by a national corporation. The corporation was looking for someone to market the facility, and I was looking for a way to move up the ladder. The director of nursing believed I had good public relations skills, and she asked me if I thought I could market the nursing home. I said I could. I knew that the business end was important because of the emphasis on competitiveness in health care today. I wanted to be prepared for the business aspects, so I took the marketing job.

Some believe that calloused people with low skills are hired to work in nursing homes. That isn't true. There are some excellent people giving care in those homes. My job was to interpret that fact for the public.

I brought my nursing knowledge to the marketing job. I could set up programs—such as outpatient kidney dialysis in the nursing home—and also teach the staff the procedures. Most marketing people are business people and not professional nurses. With my health care background, I understood the clinical as well as the business problems. I decided that if I was to get anyplace in health care administration, I'd need to understand the fiscal situation better, so I went on for my master's in Business Administration. It's taken me three years, and I plan to finish my degree this spring.

I learned a lot about business that other nurses don't always appreciate or understand. Sometimes, with the federal regulations, certain stipulations are placed on health care agencies that cause real ethical problems for the people working there. For instance, it is important to have a certain "payer mix" if the health facility is going to stay in the black. Private patients subsidize the cost of patients on Medicare, so you need to reduce the Medicare admissions and increase the private payers. That's hard to do, because you have to turn away some needy patients on Medicare.

I loved the job. I was learning a lot and I felt that I was really giving a valuable service. The only time the staff bucked me was when I wanted to bring respirator patients into the nursing home. This was more than they wanted to deal with—some respirator patients have very complex needs; others are very simple to care for. After all, families take care of people on respirators in their own homes.

The staff's resistance posed a dilemma for me. I was hired to market the institution. Caring for respirator patients was a needed service and an excellent way to increase revenue. I went to the president with the hope of gaining his support. Eventually, it became a sort of power struggle as to who was going to have the say, the staff nurses or me. I was slowly edged out of product development, so I left.

My time in the marketing job was well spent. I had made contacts, and I was well known, particularly in long-term care. I then went into consultation, doing proposals for acute care hospitals that wanted to start a long-term care facility.

Shortly afterward, I was contacted by my present employer, the director of the state mental health hospital. The mental health hospital still has a stigma. It needs good public relations by someone who can appreciate the good things being done here and can tell the public about it. State mental hospitals are very political systems. I've learned more about politics and how to effect change through the use of the political system. If I had known how to effect change better when I was in nursing, I probably would have stayed in it.

I'll stay in this kind of job as long as I can continue to be involved in developing new programs. That's how I use my nursing background. I would not stay in marketing if I could not have an influence on the product I'm selling. After all, that's the reason I didn't stay in nursing.

29

Offering the Elderly an Alternative

Elaine's small office, in the back of a converted storefront, gives little indication of the million-dollar alternative-living enterprise she directs. Elaine is a dropout from institutional nursing. After a two-year hiatus, she found a way to practice independently and use her community nursing skills on behalf of the elderly

I'd worked in a two-hundred-and-seventy-bed nursing home, and I was supposed to coordinate the education of all the professionals and aides employed there. I ended up being plugged in . . . wherever. I left because I was frustrated.

I decided I wouldn't work anymore. I had money, so I didn't need to work, but I became bored. I took a part-time job with a home care agency, and I was working there when an opportunity came up.

My husband is in real estate. A hospital administrator friend called him to say that he knew a man who wanted to sell a small group home for the elderly. He suggested we go into partnership with him and run it. His wife was an activities director at a nursing home, and he felt that the pooled knowledge and experience of the four of us would lead to a good partnership.

Six months later, we were starting our first group home. For me, it originally was going to be a part-time job—a sideline to complement my home care job. That was three years ago—we're opening our seventh home this spring.

We thought running an alternative living home would be a breeze. In the beginning, we hired a cute little couple as independent contractors, and we tried to make it very simple, as far as fringe benefits go. We soon learned that you can't run it as a "ma and pa" operation—it wasn't going to work. We now have over fifty employees, and we cover their unemployment, workman's compensation, and health insurance packages.

We're the independent contractor now. I've had to hire three nurses. The state requires that we monitor the health care of every resident. Each resident is seen at least once a month by the nurse, just to go over any existing health problems or to answer any questions they may have about their doctors' visits, medications, and so forth. We have nursing care plans for all of our fifty-six residents.

Many elderly don't need to be in nursing homes; they just need some supervision, though not necessarily from a nurse. On the other hand, many of the people I used to see in home care really needed more supervision than what they were getting by having an aide or nurse come into their homes once or twice a week. The elderly people would fall apart between visits. They really needed daily supervision, but the cost was prohibitive. We thought a group home would be a perfect setting. The elderly would receive twenty-four-hour, around-the-clock supervision at a reasonable cost.

A non-nurse could not do my job. I determine which residents will move into the house and which ones will not. I also make the final decision when it's time for someone to move out. My three partners show the homes to prospective families just as much as I do, but they always consult me when they decide someone can move in. My partners don't even know the right questions to ask.

They make the right decisions from the facts, but I'm skilled at finding out little things that the families don't always mention voluntarily. For instance, a daughter might say, "Mama can't find her way to the bathroom at night." The cues me to question if she is incontinent or unable to tolerate laxatives, has a vision problem, or is disoriented at night.

No matter what the health problem, as long as the resident can handle it independently, she may live in the home. We will take people with colostomies. I have not had a request for someone with an in-dwelling catheter, but I wouldn't rule it out. We like to take people who are continent—or, if they are incontinent, we want them to be able to handle it themselves. We don't need to be responsible for cleaning them up.

Some of our clients have no apparent health problems. I once tried to talk a man out of moving into the home. I think it was his eightieth birthday that triggered his request to move in with us. He'd been living in a duplex, he had his own car, and he went to a meal site every day. He had a routine of activity. He didn't want to take meals with us because his friends were at the meal site. He wanted a refrigerator in his room, which we allowed him to have. So he had juices, hard-boiled eggs, fruit, bread, and sandwiches, and he took his other meals out. I thought that, after a while, the home-cooking smells would get him to change his mind, but they never did. He was with us a year and four months, and he went out every single day. He didn't participate in any activities with the residents. A couple of times, I offered him just the room, because he was paying a lot for staying in the home and not using any of our services, but he said, "No, I want to be here in case I get sick." A few months ago, one of his meal-site friends lost his wife, so our resident decided to move in with his friend. I think when he turned eighty, he was just afraid something was going to happen and he felt he shouldn't be living alone. He couldn't find a rooming house that was suitable for him. With us, he knew someone was always there.

All of our residents are private pay; there is no outside funding. If the government paid for this type of care, we would be deluged. Instead, the government pays for nursing home care which is much more expensive and not as good. Alzheimer patients in nursing homes don't have two staff for eight people, as we do.

We have three homes designed specifically for residents with Alzheimer's, for people who will never return to independent living. You could never run Alzheimer homes without nurses. Either myself or our nurse consultant is in each Alzheimer home at least once a week because of the inability of some of the residents to express their physical problems. If we weren't doing this, the staff would be calling doctors every day. The staff working with Alzheimer residents go through a formal training program conducted by nurse gerontologists. They learn things to watch for, the signs of distress the residents aren't able to vocalize. The staff also get an hour-and-a-half orientation that I teach. They learn what to do in nonemergency situations, such as when a resident is running a fever, and they learn a series of steps to take before they call a nurse. We talk about pain, bodily discomfort, and how it might be expressed. When the staff do call me or the other nurses, they have their little piece of paper out that describes the pulse, respiration, where the pain is, and so on. For the most part, staff call the doctors themselves. They're the ones with the residents; they're the ones who should be trained to talk with the doctors or the residents' families.

Good doctors—who are familiar with the health problems of the elderly—are difficult to find. When I have the opportunity, I'll recommend a nearby geriatric center to the families. We nurses communicate mostly through the nurses there. All the physicians at the center are pretty good. They do listen and know what drugs are appropriate for elderly patients. We've had physicians in other clinics who ignored our resident complaints or prescribed drugs inappropriately. I still have trouble finding eye doctors and dentists who are good with the elderly.

There has been a lot of community resistance to some of our homes, but it's becoming less so. We're still in court with the Maple Grove suburb. A nurse headed up the opposition. It was personally very embarrassing to me that she was a nurse, especially after the crazy things that she said. She had a neighborhood meeting and said, in front of twelve people, that the Franklin Park Alzheimer Home had bars on the windows. She didn't have the facts. Usually, neighborhood opposition is not directed at us personally. The main opposition is to the fact that once a house is licensed for community residential, if we choose to move and sell out, other groups that the community sees as less desirable can move in. The communities want a deed restriction and, from a business standpoint, we can't do that.

I've hired the nurses in our business as independent contractors. I explain that they're hired to do a job and they'll make the same amount of money whether the job takes five hours or five days. It all depends on their efficiency.

One thing they stressed in my master's program at the university was to go out and make a job for yourself, create a role in the community that wasn't there before. There are many opportunities for other nurses in this kind of business—if they want to create their own jobs. A few years ago, people laughed when I talked about creating their own business opportunities. I can't tell you how many referrals I'm getting now from nursing homes. Patients enter nursing homes under Title XIX, which only pays for a high level of skilled care, and when the patient no longer requires that level of care or ceases to progress, the government stops paying. The patients have nowhere to go.

Another problem group are people living in life care centers. These are places where people contract to be taken care of for life. Initially, they're in independent living quarters, but eventually they need to be moved to the nursing home where they require skilled care much longer than was anticipated. The nursing home beds of these life care centers are full, and they need to move some residents out.

Right now, I have two of these people, funded by the state. We don't want to count on this, however—it's limited funding that's not guaranteed. I can't tell a family that it's okay to have the father or mother move into our house, but when the money runs out we can't keep them.

I don't know where all these people are going to go. Most are in their eighties. They don't want to live alone, even when they can have community services brought in—services such as Meals-on-Wheels. They prefer not to be in an institution, but without a lot of money, where are they going to go?

30

Nurse Practitioner Turned Rolfer

Mary is a nurse who uses touch for healing. Her office is on the second floor of a defunct grade school building.

I can't say that I've given up nursing. Instead, rolfing [a body alignment technique developed by Dr. Ida F. Rolf, a physiologist] provides the best way to practice for me. It allows me to use all my skills. I can use my hands for the good of another. That may sound funny, but that's why I came into nursing. Doing something, physically, for people is extremely important to me.

Prior to becoming a rolfer, I had several jobs in nursing. I'd been a staff nurse, and I'd done some teaching in public health, so my experience was pretty broad. From 1975 to 1981, I was a nurse practitioner.

In the late seventies, I was involved in self-fulfillment experiences, such as gestalt therapy. I got rolfed. I knew then that I would someday do rolfing myself. I saw it as a way to have client contact, as well as a means of getting away from the dominance of the medical profession.

Rolfing is total body therapy work. The rolfer sees the body, mind, and spirit of the client connected. I'm not saying that this is the therapy—that's not true. It's hands-on work that simply balances the body in the gravitational field of the earth. That's the bottom line. However, for those clients who will allow it, some very powerful things can happen for them. Some say they are more self-confident, have greater concentration, and generally have a greater emotional as well as physical well-being.

The basic assumption in rolfing is that physical and psychological assaults occur through life that lead to unhealthy body configurations. People respond to physical and psychological stress by holding their bodies a certain way. They compensate physically. This compensation causes problems in the body alignment and, as a result, you get other problems.

For example, let's say that you have an injury to the leg that requires casting. Carting a heavy cast around for several weeks is bound to put the body out of alignment. Later on, you may have back pains because the muscles of the spine have been thrown off. Psychological stress can also have the same effect.

When a person comes to me, the first thing I do is carefully observe the way he walks, sits, stands, uses his muscles. He then lies down on a padded rolfing table. I proceed to use my hands to manipulate the connective tissue, called fascia, that covers the muscle. It's fascia that gives the body its shape. Rolfers believe that the fascia is the structure that holds the physical and emotional trauma of a person's life.

I work on that tissue, lengthening, releasing it, so the body can take its natural shape. The total process takes ten sessions. The therapy allows the person to become more of what he is completely capable of being, with little influence from me. I have an idea of how the body should look, but as you free up these structures, people assume their own postures. I don't diagnose, and I don't treat. I simply work to balance the body.

In my first job as a nurse practitioner, I worked with patients in a hypertension clinic. This was an experimental program sponsored by the Department of Preventive Medicine of a medical college. The nurse practitioners were responsible for setting up and administrating the clinic. We carried out the medical plan independently, unless there was a problem. We had a collegial relationship with the doctors.

The clinic hired nurses, rather than physicians, primarily because of cost. It was cheaper for us to do the job. We were getting a nurse's salary for doing many of the doctor's tasks. Also, Dr. Cassidy and the other men working at the clinic thought we could do a better job than the doctors. Hypertension, day after day, can be boring for physicians. Nurses who like to look at all aspects of patient care are never bored.

For about a year and a half, we had a really good collegial relationship with the docs. Then, a physician—an internist from another department—joined our department. He was appalled at what we were doing. He said, "No way should nurses be doing what you're doing." It was just an excuse to get us out—in reality, he needed the room for teaching medical students, so we were bumped from the clinics. Medical students gave free help, so he didn't need nurse practitioners anymore.

Because of the hospital union, they couldn't fire us, so the administration transferred us to the emergency room. The medical director was dismayed to lose us, but he went along with his colleagues when push came to shove.

We pleaded with the nursing supervisor to petition the union about our case, but she didn't want to create waves. She told us, "Leave things the way they are. After all, you're getting paid and you still have jobs."

A nurse colleague said, "To hell with this; if I can't beat 'em, I'll join 'em." She entered medical school and is now a practicing physician. Just to show you how chauvinistic that internist was, he told her, "Forget medical school—stay home and have kids."

That nurse had the option of going to medical school. I did not. I was a single parent with two children to support. Besides, I had taken a few courses in medical school and I knew that I didn't want to pursue medicine. I wanted to continue my nursing career.

People come to me for different reasons. Athletes, for instance, simply want to perform better, and that's exactly what has happened with every athlete I've worked with. I've had some pretty amazing things happen. One fellow had severe back problems—two slipped discs. These were giving him so much pain that he'd contemplated suicide. Prior to coming to me, he'd been through the whole medical system for a couple of years. He'd had chymopapain [an enzyme related to papain] to treat the discs. I'd worked with his sister, who was a nurse, and she suggested to him that he try rolfing. "There isn't much else you can do," she told him, "and it might help."

The man is now riding his bike fifty miles at a time. He lifts one-hundred-pound weights. He is more pain-free than he ever imagined he could be. He recently saw his physician, who said, "You certainly have changed dramatically," and he said, "That's because I've been rolfed," The physician shook his head and said, "No, such results couldn't be due to rolfing. You took longer than normal to respond to the chymopapain treatment, that's all." Actually, he was way past the time when anyone has been known to respond to chymopapain.

That's a dramatic example. Others get rid of aches and pains, increase their mobility. Take the elderly—after rolfing, they're balanced better, and they walk better.

I work with babies and children. I see kids whose legs are turning in. The goal there, obviously, is to strengthen their legs. It's gratifying to see the shape of their legs change. You know their lives are going to go a whole lot differently.

Last month, I completed rolfing a woman executive who was under a lot of stress. She'd complained of debilitating headaches. She has been headache-free ever since. I recently rolfed a lady with temporomandibular joint (TMJ) problems. What happens is people grind down on their teeth and the jaw gets tight at the hinge. If this condition persists, nerves are pressed and terrible pain occurs. This woman's dentist wanted her to wear a plate in her mouth at night. She refused. Now, after rolfing, her dentist is surprised to find her jaw much more relaxed.

Lately, I've been working with handicapped children. There is some interesting information coming out of the Rolfing Institute suggesting that rolfing can make a difference for these children. I've had some interesting results myself.

One youngster with Down's syndrome had been in physical therapy since she was five months old. Obviously, I started with a good situation. Since rolfing started, her breathing normalized. Her body tone has gone from flaccid to having some vigor. Even her language has improved. She's much more verbal, and she lets me know what she wants now. She'll point and tell me, "I want rolfing here, and I don't want you to go there." The effect of her autonomous development is unclear. We need to study these children.

I've got some other ideas for research that I would like to pursue. A nurse faculty at the university is interested in collaborating on research, and we plan to write a grant, get some money, and pursue our ideas. It's interesting how I always come back to nursing.

I would be interested in researching the effects of rolfing so I could influence the attitudes of the medical community. If rolfing could get rid of pain, why not use it before resorting to pills or drastic surgery? Physicians and nurses need to know that manipulation should be an option for patients.

Physicians whom I speak with individually are supportive of rolfing. I've not met individual resistance. Collectively, the medical society hasn't endorsed us. My physician referrals have come from those who were themselves rolfed. The problem with referrals is that rolfing isn't covered by insurance companies.

Rolfing has allowed me to use all of my knowledge to the fullest, which is something I was not able to do in the structure of the health care bureaucracy. Nurses need to recognize that they have a wide repertoire to use for healing and comforting. They do not need to be tied to medicine. They, themselves, are healers.

31

Navy Nurse

Mary Ellen's credentials are impressive. Navy commander, college professor, president of a state nurses' association, and recipient of honorary awards.

It's ironic that I'm in the Navy reserve now. Even today, people think that, because I'm in the reserve, I support all the defense spending. It's not true. It's not that I believe we should go to war—I believe that when our guys are fighting, they deserve to have good medical care. To not join because I hate war is to stick those guys with a double whammy, like Vietnam—those guys didn't want to be there, either.

I've been in the Navy ten years now, and I've never been on a ship. The one time we were scheduled to tour a ship, there was a hurricane the night before. All ships were put out to sea, without us, to prevent hurricane damage.

Navy nursing certainly is different than civilian nursing. In the Navy, the nurses run things and the physicians know it. The old staff cues in the new physician recruits. They tell the new guys, "The nurses are the ones who will make or break you, so you'd better watch what you're doing."

We had no prima donnas on our wards, no physicians throwing fits like you'll see in civilian hospitals. That wasn't allowed. If a doctor got feisty, the nurse took care of him and he never did it again.

This was the case in the emergency room, too. One time, a doctor was doing a procedure and he started yelling at the nurses. They told him, "We don't talk that way around here. We'll come back when you clean up your act, when you can talk to us like an adult." Zoom! They were gone! The doctor was left trying to do a procedure by himself. You better believe the doctors quickly learned what was acceptable and what wasn't.

After officers' training in '72, they asked me where I wanted to work. I said my specialty was pediatrics. Military nurses didn't go into peds, so I ended up on orthopedics. Ortho was where I met Ms. Crane, a crusty lieutenant commander who fit the stereotype of the old service nurse. Still, when you scratched the surface of Crane, you found a very complex, caring person.

For instance, fellows coming from overseas had no money. Their possessions, including their pay records, had been scattered to the four corners of the earth. A lot of the guys were casted, and the amputees were fitted with pylons. Neither the military nor the Red Cross supplied these guys with shoes. Without them, they might lay around in bed for weeks. With shoes, they'd be home in ten days. Well, I discovered Ms. Crane in the military exchange one day, buying shoes for these guys with her own money.

That's when I started to take a different look at her. She *needed* to be stern. She was dealing with corpsmen who were seventeen to nineteen years old. We all were brand-new nurses, wet behind the ears.

Ms. Crane was an enigma. I remember going to her house and being overwhelmed at the beauty of her furnishings. Here was this very austere, military lady with all these beautiful dainty things. She'd been all over the world during her military career—Italy, Spain, Japan. Her house was full of fine glass, china, lace tablecloths.

During my stint in the emergency room, I did night duty. At nighttime, the emergency was closed, so you were rotated to the open-heart ward. I knew zilch about the care of open-heart surgery patients. We had patients of all ages, sixteen months and up. I was scared to death. The thing that saved me—and the patients—was that surgery was done on Tuesdays, Wednesdays, and Thursdays. On each of those nights, the resident slept on a sleeper sofa and was readily available when I got in trouble. That's the only thing that kept me sane. By the weekend, the patients were in pretty good condition and I could manage without the resident. I liked being a Navy nurse. We were given a lot of responsibility and the wherewithal to deal with it. In comparing notes with my civilian friends, I found that I learned faster and was moved up the ladder faster than the civilian nurses. I felt comfortable handling emergencies.

You learned to survive. Service people have developed a bartering system they call "come shawing." When you are come shawing, you're going after something you need but have no legitimate way of requisitioning. When I was working in the emergency room, one of the photographic services fellows came in requesting a glass thermometer. I traded him two glass thermometers for six glossy black-and-white photos of the nurse corps' birthday party.

We tried to empty out the wards for the holidays. We had about eight to ten guys and their girlfriends on the ward for one New Year's Eve. This group was ready for a party. Somebody had brought in a stereo. We had food galore, hors d'oeuvres, and cold duck. You weren't supposed to have wine, so we hid the cold duck in brown bags. The place was booming, streamers all over the place, food and drink, music blaring.

Out of the corner of my eye I saw Ms. Crane coming. I thought, "Oh, oh, if she's going to yell at me, it had better not be in front of everyone." I started to walk toward her. She was within three feet of me and had this grim look in her face. "Turn *down* the music," she said to me and, with that, she turned on her heels and walked out.

She usually made second rounds about eight-thirty at night. This night, she didn't come back until much later. By that time, these guys were all out like a light. The fellows were all on Valium as muscle relaxants, and Valium plus cold duck *really* relaxed them.

We took care of a lot of V.I.P.'s—even the president. Nobody is supposed to know the location of the presidential suite, but everybody does. I didn't have the status, but several of my friends took care of President Nixon.

A lot of chaos is created when a V.I.P. such as the president is admitted. His staff literally takes over the hospital. Our regular switchboard operators have to step aside for the White House communications staff. Now, this is a thousand-bed hospital, we are winding down from Vietnam, so we're packed and here comes the White House communications staff to *run* our switchboard.

The Secret Service took over all kinds of stuff—blocked the stairwells. All the P.M. nurses' parking spots went to the Secret Service. It made all the nurses mad.

The other thing about the Navy was the personal relationships we developed. Here we were, essentially all just out of adolescence, dealing with heavy stuff. We'd get together a lot outside of work, doing group things, having holiday dinners. We went to parties with patients. You were like family to them, especially when they had no family. It didn't interfere with the patient relationship, but it did cause problems when these guys died.

People in the community were good to us and the men. Sometimes they got carried away. We'd get carloads of funeral flowers to "brighten up" the wards. Funeral arrangements are distinctive. Nobody who is in the hospital wants to be reminded of funerals. During the quiet hours, the nurses would take the flowers to the utility room and rearrange them. We became very creative in flower arrangement! The guys got a big charge out of our antics; half of them knew what we were doing.

I can't think of anything really bad to say about the service. I got out of active duty for only one reason—the chief nurse was about to retire. Her replacement and I didn't hit if off at all. I volunteered to reenlist if I could get out of Bethesda. I volunteered to go to Adak, Alaska. I volunteered to go to Greenland. That's how desperate I was to get away from the replacement chief nurse. The military said that I'd probably get transferred, but that wasn't good enough for me. I'd had a previous experience in which I waited over a year for a transfer out of the E.R. —and that time, the transfer was *guaranteed.* When I heard the word "probably," I said. "No way." If that lady became the chief nurse, I'd have probably wound up in the kitchen before they got around to transferring me out. I left active duty.

Sometimes I miss active duty. I can't take it like I used to, though. Active reserves pretty near killed me last summer. We had to get up this steep hill. I wasn't sure I'd make it. While we were on maneuvers, a fellow fell down climbing the mountain and had a concussion. We went up and got the kid. I was in the back of the truck, holding this kid while the driver was whizzing down this mountain. During those times, I miss active duty. Thankfully, the feeling passes quickly.

PART SEVEN

MOVERS AND SHAKERS

Among the ranks of nurses are those who use exceptional talents to challenge the status quo. These strong nurses won't tolerate artificial barriers to their practice rights—they imagine the future and fulfill their own prophecies. Movers and shakers get their piece of the pie through political savvy, knowledge of economic imperatives, grantsmanship, and marketing strategies. They are nurses who selflessly labor to better the status of the profession and quality of patient care.

As we've seen throughout this book, these are concerns shared by most nurses, yet few are in the position—or willing to place themselves in the position—to take an active stance in creating change. The three nurses in this section have done so.

"It's up to us as individuals to make it happen," advises Sheila, a woman who made her career choices late in her life. Her political acumen, honed through years of work in the Democratic Party, proved quite useful when she landed a position on a medical college board, where she is using her status to initiate important changes that will affect nursing in the future.

For Dean Shannon, the way for nursing to gain prominence is for nurses to show the difference they can make in patient outcomes. This can be done only when nurses control their practice settings. Dean Shannon believes nurses must act to shape their own future and not wait for permission. Not one to merely give lip service to her philosophy, her deeds show she is a woman of action.

On a more general plateau, there is the matter of quality assurance. Dean Jensen, whose scholarship has led to the creation of a model for quality assurance, argues that it is not enough to simply assess *the quality of patient care, it is a matter that has to be* assured, *for the benefit of both patients and nurses. It is to this goal that she devotes her efforts.*

Politics in nursing, like politics in general, is a complex undertaking that moves at a very slow pace. For many, the lack of immediate results is intimidating or discouraging. For others, like the three voices in this section, the politics of nursing issues a challenge that cannot go unheeded.

32

Making It Happen

At first glance, it's hard to believe that Sheila has a son in college—cocktail waitresses still ask her for her I.D. Petite and composed, she wears a classic tweed suit. For Sheila, nursing wasn't a career choice made early in life.

I really had no career at all until I'd spent ten or fifteen years at home. After high school, I went to a private college, spent two years as a biology major, quit, got married, and had three children. In my last five years at home, I'd gotten to know my friend Barbara. She was an emergency room nurse at the time. She absolutely loved emergency care. When it came time for me to look at a career of my own, I chose nursing. Barbara had shown nursing to be a very exciting occupation and career—though I didn't want to go into emergency room nursing. Too much blood and guts for me.

I decided on a four-year baccalaureate program. I already had sixty credits and some science. When I showed them my transcripts, there was a fair amount of resistance from the director of the program. It was very clear to me that they were putting up stumbling blocks. I'm not sure why they were so resistant to someone who obviously had done well academically.

On the other hand, the two-year associate degree program was eager to have me. They seemed to value me as an individual and potential nurse. I went that route, knowing full well it would just take me longer to get that BSN.

I guess I feel somewhat messianic about women and about nurses in particular. Nurses are a group of women who don't have enough self-confidence to get what they need from this world. It's as broad as that. At one point, I wasn't confident, either. But change can happen with people and with groups. It's very exciting when those changes actually happen.

We nurses have some very strong opponents—or adversaries, if you will—in terms of the medical community. Physicians feel they own the turf. That was very clear when we tried to pass the new Nurse Practice Act. Physicians have no concept of what nursing diagnosis is. They feel that the world "diagnosis" is theirs! They don't even understand that their car mechanics will diagnose what's wrong with their cars.

Part of it is a turf issue—they're *unwilling* to understand. It's also an economic thing. Physicians are having problems under DRGs, with people dictating to them how they will practice. When they learned that nurses wanted to insert nursing diagnosis in the Nurse Practice Act, they figured this is one thing they could curtail.

So we nurses have our work cut out for us in the state, if we intend to pass a practice act that will speak to an image of nursing that is current and relevant, that is an alternative for the public. And it may take another biennium to get it accomplished. It may take time after that as well. People get discouraged. They say, "We took them a package and it didn't work." I personally think we are in a much better position than we were a year ago.

I was one of the founding members of a group in Rock County called the Democratic Women's Campaign Association. It was founded on the premise that women have a much more difficult time getting funds to run for public office than men do—that women, by and large, are more apolitical than men are. The group was organized to help educate the public and help raise funds for women candidates.

We've been fairly successful. We had Gloria Steinem in

for wonderful kinds of events. We had the lady with the hat —Bella Abzug, from New York. We raised maybe $20,000 in the course of four years with fund-raising events.

One committee focus gets women more involved politically, helps them find areas of influence. We get a printout from the State Democratic Party office of all the boards and commissions the Governor makes appointments to. When these different appointments are coming up, we've been successful in getting many of our members appointed.

I'd really never been all that involved in politics in New York, where I'd come from. I moved to Springfield in 1969. Shortly after I moved, I registered to vote. Soon after, I got a call from Joan Matthews, who is now our congressional district representative in Washington. She asked me if I wanted to be a precinct committee person. I told her that I didn't know what that meant. She said, "Why don't you come over to the house and we'll talk about what that means." So I did.

I soon found myself a precinct committee person and, through Joan, I got heavily involved within the Democratic Party in Rock County. By virtue of the lack of females around, I found myself a member of the scholarship committee, then chair of scholarship. I was also a member of the screening committee for candidates seeking public office, and then I was chairperson of that committee.

Since 1970, I've taken an active role in the Democratic Party's processes in Rock County. That has always been interesting, helpful, and fun. In 1980, I went as a delegate to the national convention. That, of course, was fantastic. In 1984, I was asked to chair the Central Committee.

I lecture to almost all the schools of nursing in the Springfield area. I talk to the students about taking an active role in politics. I try to make that as easy for them to understand as I can. I use the analogy that even the decision a family makes about where they're going to go on vacation is a political decision. Every member has an idea about where he or she wants to go, but there is only enough money for one vacation. So everyone jockeys to be the first in line, or present the best case or what have you. Politics is really no different from that.

I tell the students that political people make decisions about how they live their lives, from as simple a decision as to whether they get their garbage picked up to a decision as complex as what kind of Nurse Practice Act they'll have in their state. What the act is like, how they can practice, the relationship between physicians and nurses—those kinds of things—are all decided in the political arena. Whether the nurses sit on policy-making boards or are on boards of trustees is decided by political people. To remove yourself from the political process means that you play "left out."

I lobbied for three years for the position as trustee on the board of the medical college in Springfield. I did it for three years, knowing full well that, as a student in a nursing program, I wasn't going to be appointed. But that was all right—it just takes time. I think that sometimes nurses just don't understand that it takes two or three attempts at doing something before it's not a shock anymore. The governor appointed me as a trustee last year.

The president and three other board members were dead set against my appointment to the board. I found that out afterward. But the governor had already made his decision and was not going to back down. The majority of the board members are business people. There are nine members, all appointed by the governor. Before I joined, there was a token woman.

At the first board meeting I attended, everyone was polite. They said, "Welcome," of course. Then we had dinner. One of the board members, who was less than socially astute, came up to the member on my right and said, "See? She's not going to be so difficult to get along with." If there had been a hole, this guy would have fallen into it! It showed me that they'd been thinking, "What are we going to do with this person?" They feared I was going to disrupt their whole arena.

I'd spent some time with a retired female faculty member who had been on the board of trustees at our university. I asked her how she made sure she wasn't perceived in an antagonistic way. I learned that she really hadn't been that successful. She'd been walled off.

I thought, "You can't be successful if you're walled off and everybody agrees with what you suggest, when what you're suggesting doesn't go anywhere. I can't have that happen. I've got to play this very low key for a period of time. I'll just ask questions."

There is no way you can come in as a firebrand or a crazy person. They would just write you off, and you're only one of nine. I have to structure the nine years in such a way that achieves a crescendo effect in terms of accomplishments. Build those liaisons, do your groundwork, gain credibility. I realize that this is a nine-year appointment. This first year has been my year to ask questions, to point out inconsistencies as just an innocent kind of thing, you know. Also, I've tried to build linkage and support with the other board members in terms of the future.

After I'd been on the board three or four months and was having very little contact with the president, I decided it was about time I went to see him and really be very clear that, though I obviously had interests in nursing, I was not so foolish as to be centrally focused. I mean, I have a much broader understanding.

The medical college is important to me as an entity. I told him, "I'm going to be the best board member you've ever seen. I have a lot of expertise in the political arena that many board members don't have. When you need help getting things done, I'll be there for you."

I don't know how successful I was with him, but I thought that I'd go there and say those things and have a very heart-to-heart talk with him. I think he's someone who doesn't trust people readily, so it will take time for him to believe me. He said, "I know what's happened," meaning that he knew there were members talking against my appointment. He said, "It has nothing to do with you personally."

I said, "I know that."

"It has to do with your being a nurse," he told me.

And I said, "I know that."

From his perspective, he didn't want someone being an advocate for just one portion of the medical school. In his own mind, he didn't see that there were many members already there who were solely advocates for medicine! I wouldn't say that he now holds me at arm's length. He certainly doesn't talk with me as he does the chairman, but that will come with time. He uses me to do things for him, in terms of the political arena at the state level. And that's OK. I welcome that. I do his bidding for the things that I think are important. So it works.

A physician from Stanford gave an excellent presentation to the board on the future of health care. He suggested we would be focusing on chronic kinds of diseases instead of the medical model. I was sure the board wouldn't necessarily be interested in any nursing articles, but I thought they might be interested in a physician article. I sent a copy of an article by this physician to the president of the college. For the next board meeting, he copied that article and it was at everybody's place.

See, you need to ask, "Who is the messenger?" You need to make sure the framework is in words that they can understand. Then the message will get shared; it will get through, and it will work. That was an exercise that worked. I identified that it had to come from a physician. If it had come from a nurse, he would have said, "Oh, that's nice, but . . ."

I get so upset with public relations that wants to portray all nurses in any given institution as the warm, fuzzy kind of person. P.R. doesn't even want to touch the fact that here is a critical thinker, here is somebody who can intervene for you. Here is someone who is skilled in communication and can listen to you. We may be perceived as being warm and fuzzy, but that's real skill, too, you know. Public relations doesn't want to touch that information. They want to look at a white-dressed, becapped kind of nurse and portray the caring kind of thing. That's all they want to deal with because they think that's what the public wants.

I guess I feel some responsibility in terms of public education. Yes, you give them a little bit of that because that's the lead-in. But you also give them the other kind of information that'll help them be better health care consumers.

The physician wouldn't want another image, nor do administrators, who see the physicians as their customers.

Patients really don't want another one, either. It's a situation that really isn't set up for success or making those kinds of images available to the public.

Maybe it will take nurse entrepreneurs and their own kinds of businesses, offering their alternatives, figuring out those images to portray to the public. It will probably not come out of the institutions themselves; they're too tied in to old models. It's up to us as individuals to make it happen.

33

Something of Value

Dean Shannon is the head of a midwestern university's School of Nursing. We shared a quick lunch together, during the second day of the Midwest Nursing Research Conference. Dean Shannon's softly draped jacket carries the eye down to her voluminous pantaloons nipped in at the ankles above her slipper pumps. Tailored suits seem dull in comparison. Her hair is as casually elegant as her suit; her eyes, however, reflect business and determination.

Our profession has spent twenty years fighting about educational issues—which type nurse is better, depending on her education. A total waste of time and productivity. We should have spent that time defining our clinical practice and our future. Nursing faculty for too long have concentrated on fitting into academic models by earning their way up through rank and tenure. We've forgotten we are a practice discipline, that the education and research of our professional practice needs to be our focus.

All of our faculty activities now aim to integrate these three things—education, practice, and research. I know faculty can't wear all three hats, but as a group we can.

Our School of Nursing runs a state-accredited health care agency. The majority of our patients' home visits are delivered by nursing faculty and students. We began by having faculty and students conduct home visits for a satellite physician family practice clinic.

Initially the physicians thought nurses only did what physicians told them to do. Within a year's time the physicians and residents realized that our home visits were adding tremendously to the physicians' practice. Patients began following medical orders better, their hospital admissions were reduced, they stayed healthier between clinic visits.

During the summer, the chief of family practice came to me and said, "We need to have your faculty and students seeing our patients year 'round, not just during the school year." I answered, "Well, you need to pay for them, then, because faculty are not under contract in the summer." He said, "I don't have the money."

Within a year he was back. "I have the money now," he said. By this time I had decided we should have our own clinic, so I answered, "I don't need your money; now I need your support. Let's go to the State Board of Health together; let's go to the college administration." Within six weeks we had a state-certified home health agency connected with the Family Practice Clinic.

We are not in the business of being the best home care agency in the world; we are in the business of solving the problems of the nursing profession. Faculty are delivering services, identifying their quality, checking community response, participating in marketing, asking, "How do we get referrals?" In short, we are learning to run and market ourselves as a health care business.

Once we started, the Office on Aging called to ask if we would offer a competitive bid to run wellness clinics for the elderly. Ours was the winning bid. We've set up some independent nurse-managed wellness clinics in the elderly high-rises. We learned that the elderly there do not make their own health-funding decisions; their family members do. We got their children to support us so their parents could receive the services.

We've also learned that wellness clinics in a doctor-office fashion don't work because people come in with doctor-office symptoms. Then you are dealing with illness instead of maintaining health. Wellness is something that you distribute into people's apartments, into people's lives, into classrooms.

Faculty didn't exactly stand in line saying, "Let me, take me." This is where persuasion, politicking, and arm-bending comes in. Now, five years later, gerontology has clearly become the focus of our activities. This happened not because all the faculty wanted to work in that specialty, but because they realize that the elderly are nursing's *now* population—and nursing's future.

Faculty began teaching in a long-term care facility. They grumbled about taking students there because the care was being compromised by a low nurse-patient staffing ratio. However, faculty soon became really understanding of the budget problems, costs, and Medicaid reimbursement problems. They modified a patient acuity evaluation tool for the long-term care facility. When they applied the tool, they identified that the hospital that owned the long-term care facility was transferring patients to the facility with higher acuities than the nurse-patient staffing ratio covered in the hospital.

The acuity data gave the long-term care administrator a means to negotiate for higher nurse staffing. Faculty took the same acuity data to a public hearing to get support of a separate reimbursement rate for high-intensity skilled nursing care at hospital-based, long-term care facilities.

So we influenced direct reimbursement, at least for a year or two. The hospital administrator was impressed. What could have been a threat to him suddenly became useful data that extended outside of the hospital, into the legislature. It made a direct dollar impact. Powerful, isn't it?

What we do we start quietly. There are many conservative physicians in the community. We get it started, get it working, then announce it. We found it very important to seek out the physicians who are supportive. When you have one or two physicians who are with you, other physicians don't tend to jump on you so much.

Physicians can't deny it, I mean their big concern is hanging on to their paying patients. We try to describe what we are doing as something in addition to medicine. We call and say, "This is not to threaten your practice. What we want to do is send the elderly to you more appropriately, with more useful information, because we've been working with them."

The physicians were OK. They didn't raise Cain. My contention on this—and I don't say it very often publicly—is that nursing and medicine have different publics to serve. Sometimes it's the physician who needs to be convinced of this the most.

We have submitted another proposal for a nurse-managed osteoporosis clinic. We have a faculty person who is very interested in osteoporosis research and is teaming up with several physician researchers. They have this little—it's a scanner, for want of a better description—that measures bone density of the wrist. Physicians everywhere are buying them like crazy, putting them in their offices. The physicians are able to charge a fee for saying, "Well, on a scale of one to ten, you fit here."

Nurses know that the answer to osteoporosis rests in prevention. Once it's diagnosed, therapy only helps a little. Prevention rests on early detection, thorough assessment of nutrition, exercise, activity levels, lifestyle. That's nursing. We want an osteoporosis center in the community that is set up to prevent osteoporosis, in addition to maintenance once an early diagnosis occurs. Get into high schools, get to young women. Does that give you the flavor?

We have never put the nature of our work into the values that society relates to today—special expertise, cost effectiveness, and so forth. The public shouldn't have to buy us because we are good people and care very much. We've got to deliver. We have to be able to clearly describe the outcomes of our care. The healing, the quality of life we preserve, the functioning we help the patient recover, the rawness of the illness we attenuate, the knitting together of families who have been disturbed by a member's illness. I mean, illnesses are a psychosocial, emotional, and lifestyle dysfunction as much as they are a physiological dysfunction.

We have to sell our preventive services to the publics

who are concerned about dollar costs. When we nurses can demonstrate savings through prevention, the hospitals are interested, the Feds are interested, industry is interested. If physicians aren't, there are some legislators who are. So we have to make alliances with different publics, plain and simple—alliances based on the value of our worth.

Nursing's primary initiative should be keeping people out of institutions. Our functions, the very nature of what we do is designed to do that. We already have the knowledge and skills. There is no other profession as prepared as we are for this emphasis. We need to own that and move into that role. Even when nurses are caring for elderly persons in long-term care facilities they are saving money by *preventing* decubiti [bed sores] and all that those involve.

We're missing opportunities because we do what people see us doing as opposed to what we believe we ought to be doing. There's a chasm between our values and beliefs and the way we practice.

There are ways we should more directly deal with patients. I heard a research study this morning which identified that psychiatric patients who use weekend passes do not know these visits are intended to evaluate their ability for discharge—that it is a transition mechanism—an opportunity to test their functioning, independence, ability to deal with family. The majority of patients thought it was just sort of a social activity, and so did their nurses. So where are we? Those psych nurses should be communicating, evaluating, telling patients what they can anticipate, what they should be striving for. Are the nurses not sure of the value of this?

I don't know. I just think we acquiesce too often to the external pressures. We need to ask, "What *can* we be doing?" and not be limited by institutional values.

Our faculty are talking with the HMO people. Our home health agency is contracting to do home services for the HMO. HMOs are interested in making money. They aren't going to make money if they keep adding physicians. I've suggested, "Use nurse practitioners in each of the industrial sites, for screening and health promotion activities."

And their physicians tell me—even the dean of medicine—"Oh, they cost too much, they cost more than our family practice physicians." I said, "Prove it to me."

That's what I've tried to do with our faculty. First of all, give witness to the belief that we should foster and build opportunities. We should be shaping our future rather than waiting for somebody to give us permission, rather than waiting for someone to figure out how to fund us. We have to figure out those things ourselves. Faculty and students have merged the theory of "what ought to be" with "what is." Having some ownership in the real world, they have taken the opportunity to improve it. It has made our education better, too. We show instead of tell; before, we tended to lecture too much.

Enrollment in nursing schools is declining, not only because of demographics, but because there is not a lot of esteem in our profession. There is a lot of doom and gloom. Until we take pride in what we do and know our own value and worth, we can't convince others.

You know, I talk entrepreneurial and I talk business, value, and worth, but the troubling thing is that the essence of nursing is really a holistic approach to patients. It really is the brokenness—that rawness of the human spirit—that nurses oftentimes do everything for, with, and about. I don't know if we will ever be able to measure or put a price on that.

34

Quality Is in the Eye of the Beholder

Dean Jensen's day is frequently one long string of meetings. Her husband and two teenagers absorb her discretionary time. We were fortunate to find an early morning hour free for breakfast. Her rich laugh and expansive gestures are captivating, and her intensity, as she discusses the reason for the nursing shortage, lingers after she speaks.

Quality assurance is dear to my heart. In 1973, for my dissertation, I developed a model for quality assurance in nursing. I tested that model with pediatric nurse practitioners in Wisconsin. It was kind of on the cutting edge, both because of the quality assurance topic and because pediatric nurse practitioners were beginning to work in an area nurses hadn't worked in before.

I got the idea because I was working in our state's Regional Medical Program at the time—RMPs were part of President Johnson's "Great Society." They were highly idealistic; everyone thought that if you just spread the money and the medical technology around in the right places, everybody could have the top level of care. De Bakey had done the first heart transplant, there seemed no end to the possibilities. RMPs began by funding application of medical research findings, establishing support services, and fostering cooperative health planning.

At that same time, it was the end of the Sputnik era. All

the systems people, who had put their energies into getting rockets into space, came into the health care arena. They said that health care could be a lot better if it was measured, quantified, and planned for, in the same way that you plan to put people on the moon. The engineers said that quality controls should be built into the health care system.

The RMPs picked up on this and helped people figure out how to deal with these quality issues. I happened to be working in that environment. Needless to say, I began asking. "How does this work for nursing?"

Actually, Florence Nightingale is given credit for doing quality assurance way back in the 1850s. During the early Crimean War experience at Scutari, she established quality standards that were fairly basic. She told the generals, "Our soldiers are in more danger from being in a hospital than if they were fighting on the battlefield. You'd better shape this up." They did. Later, Nightingale's recommendations for hospital management were based on her meticulously tabulated statistics on the outcomes of hospitalized patients.

In a nutshell, that's what quality assurance is all about. You figure out what you think you want, go out and measure what you have, and then take action. Unfortunately, quality assurance in the health field right now is ninety percent political and ten percent methodological—maybe even higher politically. The federal government Diagnostic Related Groups and Professional Review Organizations controls consumption of health resources, and calls it quality assurance.

Quality is what patients want to receive and what nurses want to give in terms of nursing care. Some of it is measurable, some is not. The part that is measurable usually fits into some kind of standard or criterion. For instance, a criterion measure for a patient in congestive heart failure may be to maintain adequate circulation and ventilation. It could be measured by the ventricular heart rate, respiration rate, presence of ankle edema, or presence of cyanosis.

In order to have assurance, there is another step. You know what you want in quality, and you have some way of measuring it. You measure it and *then* you take some steps to assure that the public receives this kind of care.

A lot of people want to drop the assurance part. They just don't want to be responsible or accountable for assuring quality, especially given the current cost restraints. So, in Federal Professional Review Standards, you see the words "quality assessment" used instead of "assurance." This means we only check to see if we have or have not met standards. If we haven't, remedial actions aren't assured. Professional Review Organizations are supposed to be accountable for quality. What they do is pick two or three commonly seen medical diagnoses and look at the kind of medical care that goes into this type of patient. No explicit nursing is considered.

If you look at the quality assurance model that I developed, the first step is value clarification—what is it that we value in the health care system? Right now, cost containment, competition, equal access, and quality collide. What we value is like a political football being kicked back and forth.

Nurses are getting caught in a whole lot of this. Nurses have a notion of what they believe to be quality of care, and yet the system's setup isn't necessarily conducive to carrying out that quality. The institution's cost-cutting works against it.

When nurses design their quality assurance systems, most of their criteria measure very comprehensive patient-care factors. They set forth nursing actions that will have the patient somewhat independent when he leaves the hospital. For example, the nurses will set written standards that the diabetic patient will be able to give his own insulin, take care of his feet, adjust his diet. Now, under DRGs, the physician might not admit a person to the hospital for diabetes in the first place. Or, the patient may be out before the nurses have a chance to do any of the teaching they value. All this fast "in-and-out" leaves nurses very, very concerned that people are going home without knowing how to take care of themselves.

These people are inevitably going to run into problems —even the possibility of coming back into the health care system worse off than they were before. Right now, we don't have a lot of research data to show this.

Dr. Dean, president of the American Association of Peer Review Organizations, says that quality is assumed. People think that when you cut costs, quality will still be there. It's not true. But there's little data. The people cutting costs don't necessarily want data.

On the other hand, I can become schizophrenic about nurses' quality assurance. From Florence Nightingale's time right up until today, we've conducted thousands of studies in nursing. We've developed stacks of standards. I have huge boxes just bulging with standards. Yet, I'm not sure that what we have in them helps us to understand the problems in quality *achievement.*

Frequently, the data from chart audits will show one hundred percent achievement in quality standards. On the other hand, when you talk to people who have been in the hospital lately—or, whose brothers or husbands and so forth have been in the hospital recently—you will hear the most appalling stories. Where is the discrepancy between what we hear from the people who sit down and tell us about quality, and the standards we've set?

One possibility may be that the nurse doesn't ask the patients what outcomes *they* expect to achieve. Nor do nurses document a whole lot of the patients' or families' responses to the care. Also, we retrospectively audit the standardized patient record to see whether the quality criteria have been met. The charts document only certain kinds of things. For example, the chart will say the patient slept all night, but if you ask the patient, she will say she didn't sleep a wink. Everything else is assumed to have been done, so you don't really get at the heart of what might have been the problem for the patient.

Most standards nurses have are process measures. They'll say something like, "The nurse will assess the patient and arrive at a nursing diagnosis." We are just beginning to have standards that deal with the accuracy of nursing diagnoses themselves, the nursing actions they call for, and the outcomes to be expected. These are the quality issues. The more knowledgeable nurses assess and diagnose differently, and they have a large number of ways to take care of people's problems.

In my ideal scenario, the nurse in a patient encounter would identify certain patient assessment data. She would sit with the patient and feed the data into the computer, saying, "These are all the things you and I have figured out." The computer, having been programmed for all combinations of assessment factors, would suggest nursing diagnoses. The patient and nurse would then look at these and agree or disagree with the various diagnoses. "Yes, the pain does interfere with my mobility," or "No, motivation is not a problem." They would agree on the list.

Then, up on the screen would come the most common nursing interventions for the diagnoses. The nurse and patient would agree, disagree, or add to the suggestions. They would carry these out together. The projected outcomes would be there—after so many days or so many encounters. "X" should happen.

The actions and outcomes would be aggregated in the computer for hundreds of patients. The nurses on the unit could ask the computer, "What did we accomplish for our patients diagnosed as having uncontrolled pain last month?" After pulling data up, they might say, "We haven't been doing very well at all. We'd better institute some other definitive changes." This would really be an ongoing data-based clinical quality assurance program. The standard-based process measures that we have now do not give essential information about clinical practice.

We tend to look at all kinds of different factors, not at what happened when patient and nurse work together to solve the patient's health problem. Everything else going on around the nurse-patient interaction should be measured in terms of how well that collaboration went.

Quality is what happens when nurse and patient have agreed on the patient's problem and mutually agreed on what's needed to solve his problem. Everything else in health care either enhances or impedes the solution. In reality, many of our hospital systems are set up so that quality is the last thing that happens.

Take the example of the nurse who has a dehydrated

patient on an I.V. The nurse and the patient decide he can tolerate some apple juice. The physician still has the patient NPO [nothing by mouth], so the nurse has to locate the physician to get the order changed. She gets the order. There may be no juice in the refrigerator on the unit, so she has to fill out a requisition. The diet kitchen is serving supper and will not respond. Pressed for time, the nurse may not get the juice for several hours. The I.V. is extended unnecessarily. One small thing like this in the course of caring for an acutely ill patient becomes overwhelming.

So much of nursing is like that. Nurses have the knowledge and ability to judge whether to start juice or not, without having to call the physician. The systems, like dietary, have to be set up so the nurse can do her work.

You see, something has to change out there. If nurses are unleashed to practice as professionals, instead of as gofers, it will be a career that people will select. If it continues to be an occupational career . . . no. Why would anyone spend all that time and education, only to practice and be paid at the occupational level?

Last week, at our faculty meeting, someone asked the reason our enrollments are down so far. And they *are* down! I can tell you that the class we admitted in January should have been around sixty students; it's at thirty-eight. I pointed out to faculty that it's hard to make a career choice in nursing, when staff nurses the prospective student talks to say, "Good God! Don't go into nursing. They want to hire me part time so they won't have to give me fringes. I need to work a double shift because there is not enough staff. Administration tells me nurses are not to be seen or heard."

Last week, I was having dinner with a director of nursing who told me. "The nurses in my institution haven't gotten a salary increase in six years," I almost fell off my chair. The director said to me, "You know, I used to be concerned about unions coming. You know something? I'd welcome one today."

I told my faculty, "These are the realistic things in life." It's going to take all of us to make this a profession. Peter Naisbitt, who wrote *Megatrends,* says, "Hang in there and stick to your knitting. Know what your service is and deliver it." The people who know the case delivery, the essence, are the people who are going to be in demand. These are nurses.

I would still say, "Go into nursing." If I were a young person making a career choice right now, I would go for it. However, I would put myself in the best position to be competitive. I'd go for the best education and background. I would see that words like *scientist, nurse scholar, nurse practitioner, nurse executive* become commonplace in my mind.

PART EIGHT

THE AIDS CRISIS

Few medical crises have prompted as much attention—and hysteria—as the escalating number of AIDS patients in the United States over the last decade. The disease has forced the public to confront many of its fears and beliefs—at times in such a manner that it's virtually impossible to draw proper perspectives. Sue, a director of an AIDS project, says in this section, "AIDS forces passions that bring out the best and worst in people."

This is true of the nursing profession as well. Perhaps because in each individual case nursing requires combining the exact science of medicine with the human elements, served with the topspin of a nurse's values and beliefs. As we've seen, AIDS is not a condition easy to focus on. There is a big picture, with widespread, mortal ramifications, and there is the smaller picture that finds each patient struggling with his or her humanity, trying to claim dignity in graceless death. So often, the big picture elicits anger and disgust from the general public, while the smaller vision provokes pathos and sympathy.

In this section, Sue takes a clinical look at the big picture, explaining what she has learned about the disease and the treatment of its victims. When she focuses on the small picture, as when she recalls a moment spent at a gravesite with the father of an AIDS victim, the result is heartbreaking.

As a nurse who cared for a baby born with the AIDS virus, Jane found herself in a position where she had to deal emotionally with the horror and sadness of watching an innocent die, as well as the ambivalence she felt toward the infant's drug-addicted parents.

A conclusion might have been best stated by Sue, who said that "AIDS is everyone's problem."

35

The Night Sky*

Sue is the director of the Milwaukee AIDS Project, a non-profit volunteer agency.

People often ask how I got involved in working with AIDS patients. As I reflect back, I can see that it's an enigma that I'm working with the dying, because I failed an exam on death and dying when I was a junior. At the time, my favorite patient had died in my arms, and my mother was very sick and hospitalized at the Mayo Clinic. I didn't—couldn't—deal with the idea of death and dying. I was studying to be a nurse—to make people better, not to help them die. [As the conversation unfolded it, it was obvious that death no longer cows her.]

I'd worked as a volunteer in a V.D. clinic that primarily served gay men. I worked there because I really needed to learn how to draw blood, which was something they didn't teach me to do in nursing school. I learned a lot more than how to draw blood. I learned about sexually transmitted diseases. Most of all, I witnessed different lifestyles and learned to accept them.

In April 1985, I became the director of the Milwaukee

* This interview was recorded in December 1987. Therefore, some of the theoretical material regarding the disease AIDS may be out of date.

AIDS Project. The project started in response to the needs of AIDS patients who were abandoned and had no other resources. When we started, we had a dozen volunteers, a desk, and a waiting room. Boxes were piled all around us. Our budget was about $18,000, and we had one AIDS patient.

Today, we have six paid staff, five hundred volunteers, a budget of over $400,000, and fifty AIDS patients, ranging in age from ten months to sixty-nine years. The AIDS project has two major functions—prevention education and supportive care. We run a hot-line service, a library service, provide care in the home, and hook people up with needed resources.

AIDS is everyone's problem. If you are not infected with the virus, you'll be affected. We haven't prepared ourselves for that. You may think, "AIDS won't affect me, I'm not in a risk group; I'm not gay; an I.V. drug user, or a hemophiliac, so I don't need to worry." It's simply not true. You will be affected, if not directly, then indirectly.

It no longer matters if you're gay or not. It *does* matter if you have sex with someone who is infected. Right now, AIDS isn't specific to one socioeconomic group, though it's predicted that, eventually, it will be centered among the poor. We have no idea how many people are infected or who will actually come down with AIDS. Trying to estimate the number of people infected is like looking at the night sky—the stars blink on and off faster than you can count them. Like stars cannot be seen without a telescope, Human Immunodeficiency Virus, the virus that causes AIDS, cannot be seen without a special test. That's how it is trying to estimate the number of people with AIDS. The people with AIDS now were infected years ago. So what we're seeing today are the results of activities from years ago.

It costs about forty dollars a person to test for the AIDS antibodies. It's expensive and not entirely accurate, since people could still be developing antibodies that are not picked up on the test. The tests are only for *antibodies* to the virus; we have no cost-effective way to test for the *virus* at this point. People usually develop antibodies to a virus after exposure, within six to eight weeks. With the AIDS virus, we have no guarantees. It's thought that it can be as long as six months before antibodies appear in the system.

If an antibody is found, we should assume that the person is infectious. It takes about five years for the disease to show on those who actually get AIDS. The disease is so new to this country that we don't really know the normal course of the disease.

The people who actually have the disease are a relatively small group. We have people with AIDS-related conditions, who show some but not all of the signs and symptoms of AIDS. We also have people who have the virus in their system but show no symptoms. Finally, there are those who have been exposed to AIDS, but we're not sure if they carry the virus.

For those who get it, the disease goes through several stages. I find it most useful to view AIDS in four stages in relation to nursing practice. In Stage One, the person shows antibodies. There is more and more evidence that when people are first infected, they have some type of flulike bout. If they're in the risk groups, they should be evaluated for AIDS. They may go for years—possibly ten years—without any other problems.

Night sweats are another symptom of this first stage. The sweats do not occur because the electric blanket is turned up high; it's like someone who has undergone extreme physical exertion. The mattress may be soaked through. You'll also see loss of weight—five, ten pounds without dieting. There may be increased fatigue and/or intermittent fevers. Psychosocially, the person may withdraw from social activities, and absenteeism from work may increase.

Stage Two occurs when the first opportunistic infection hits. People usually recover from this infection, but now the disease is diagnosed. As infections persist, absenteeism from work increases, which may result in loss of employment. The person probably will experience social isolation, whether it's because he feels dirty or unclean, or because he is angry and bitter. Maybe it's the first time his lifestyle has been revealed. Others may reject him because of undue fear of catching the disease.

Stage Three is when the opportunistic infections come fast and furious. The person may not recover from one infection before the next. Weight loss is extreme—frequently fifty percent of body weight. Now, the person with AIDS is truly disabled, maybe helpless. Kaposi's sarcoma are really tumors of the blood vessels, which we frequently see on the skin but which can occur anywhere. When they occur in the G.I. tract, they can cause bleeding and poor absorption of nutrients. Pneumocystic carinii pneumonia is another common opportunistic infection which causes extreme air hunger.

If patients have diarrhea associated with opportunistic infections, they may lose three to five quarts of fluid a day. We see people in different psychological phases. Some are angry, while some are unrealistically optimistic. The AIDS dementia is something that I wasn't prepared for. It's really frightening. We don't have anyone who is physically aggressive. It usually manifests itself in a patient's forgetfulness or errors in judgment. It is very difficult to differentiate dementia from substance abuse or even the normal course of grief and fear associated with a terminal illness.

In Stage Four, the individual is actively dying. We've noticed that, emotionally, there is a real switch. It depends on the nurse's rapport with the patient whether she can determine this phase. What we see are emotional closures, such as the patient's taking care of last-minute business.

Some patients refuse further treatment; others fight to the end. Pain management is important now. Patients may be confused because of the disease or the effects of the pain killers. They may be depleted of financial resources. Most of the care for these patients is nursing care, which can be managed at home. In fact, it usually can be done better at home, and it's less costly.

A major concern for nurses is infection control—to protect the patient and others. AIDS doesn't kill people; infections do. Discharge planning and providing appropriate resources is also crucial. We need to help find people to care for the patient at home. Financial help is also crucial. People with AIDS are living longer today than when I first started to work with the AIDS Project.

They need medications. These people can't afford to wait for months to get medical benefits. Treating AIDS is very expensive. The drugs used, such as AZT, only help to reduce the infections, they don't cure AIDS. AZT costs approximately $10,000 a year, and when you're unable to work and are on welfare, that's a lot of money. Since AZT is experimental, insurance companies will not cover the cost of the drug. In order to get the drug, people need to make the choice to give up their insurance and become welfare dependents. Those are pretty hard choices to make, especially when you've been self-sufficient your whole life.

Another unique phenomenon we see are the "worried well" people. They're actually not infected with HIV, but they're absolutely certain they have AIDS. They're terrorized by it. They're hysterical, they lose weight, their appetites wane, and they're fatigued—just like AIDS patients. They may need professional counseling to help them deal with their fears. AIDS isn't transmitted by casual contact. It's transmitted by blood and semen. People need to protect themselves by not letting the body fluids from another person enter their own body.

We also know that infected mothers are likely to infect their unborn babies. It's difficult to be totally certain, because you can't make a definite diagnosis of AIDS in a baby until at least one year of age.

So we see a real need for us to take a serious, mature look at our sexual practices and to communicate with our partners about our sexual practices. The sexual revolution is over. It's just too late for people to be promiscuous. Condoms are not absolute. They certainly decrease the risk, but abstinence is the only real way to prevent AIDS.

The other stereotype to break down is that AIDS only affects gay men. It's absolutely not true. It's particularly a problem in lower socioeconomic groups that share drug needles. In New York, AIDS is the major killer of women between the ages of twenty-five and thirty-five.

Actually, of all the risk populations, it's homosexual men who have been the ones to modify their sexual behavior. You may say that's a strong statement, but when you study the statistics on male rectal gonorrhea, you'll see that the rates have dropped markedly. There is only one way for men to get rectal gonorrhea and that is through homosexual activity. In contrast, the rate of cervical gonorrhea is on the rise. Since you only get cervical gonorrhea from heterosexual behavior, we know that women and heterosexual men are not practicing prevention or safer sex.

AIDS forces us to confront our feelings about homosexuality. We don't ask that anyone accept this lifestyle, but we do demand that nurses treat everyone with respect, regardless of their lifestyles. After I'd done a recent public broadcast on AIDS, I received a phone call from an irate woman quoting from the Bible about prohibitions toward homosexuality. She then finished her speech with the dirtiest, foulest language I'd ever heard, describing homosexual behavior. It was shocking. She claimed she didn't know any homosexuals and she didn't want to know them. AIDS forces passions that bring out the best and worst in people.

It also forces us to confront death, which is an uncomfortable subject in this culture. It brings us all closer to spirituality. I recall standing at the gravesite of my first AIDS patient. His father, standing next to me, was a crushed, sunken man. He said, "You know, you come into life expecting to lose your parents, and maybe even your spouse, but not your child. I don't want to leave him here. It's cold and I want to take him home just one more time. But it's too late."

Some families aren't able to deal with the dying child. Such was the case with one of my patients. John was one of the first AIDS patients we cared for. He'd left home some fifteen years before. He'd made little contact with his family during those years. He'd been a gourmet chef and a man about town. When his roommates turned him out of their apartment, he called and asked to come home. His mom said, "Sure," even though the family was unprepared to deal with the challenge of caring for a person with AIDS. John was difficult to deal with. He had little respect for others. He was careless with cigarettes and he'd spit on the floor. Finally, the parents called us and told us to come and get him and never bring him back. We literally found him and his bag on the curb.

He was pitiful. He had the skin cancer, and he'd had viral infections that affected the brain and caused personality problems. He had a colostomy and was blind in one eye. The disease had done its worst. He had no money, no medical benefits. His family had a thousand dollars in the bank. They said, "Take it—pay for his funeral and leave us alone." When you think about it, what else could they have done? They had no resources and no way to deal with him.

We had a hard time placing him. No nursing home would care for him. He wasn't near death's door, so no hospice would care for him. We looked for volunteers who would take him into their homes. He was admitted to the hospital. He lived there for months, piling up medical bills he couldn't pay. He was placed in a hospice, even though he still wasn't ready to die.

We attempted to initiate his medical benefits for months. His first check arrived after his death. AIDS challenges every system that we have. Professionals say they have never needed such extensive resources for other diseases as they have for taking care of patients with AIDS.

A good friend of mine had a very different experience. He had two opportunistic infections and that was it. He didn't have the prolonged suffering that John had. David wanted to do three things before he died—he wanted to finish his degree; he wanted to be able to leave money for his nephew's college education; and he wanted to be baptized. I recall one of our last visits when he was in the hospice. He looked very tired. I said, "People say you've given up, David." He said, "No, I haven't—I've just decided . . ." All of his personal effects were in order. Shortly before he died, he received his diploma. The day he died, one of our clergy volunteers went into the hospice and baptized him. Quietly, alone with his mother and closest friends, he turned his head on the pillow and said, "Thank you. I love you. Good-bye."

For many persons with AIDS, death is gruesome and cruel. For David it was different. Not many of us will be able to prepare for death in that way and have that sense of closure. Yes, I miss him terribly. I can no longer hug him or feel his bristly beard. But he made me understand what

I'm here for. When I thought I'd had it with this job and could no longer stand the stress, he was the person I would call. He always knew what to say. "Come on, kid, you know why you're doing this. You're doing this for people like me." And he was right. I do this because I care.

For now, care is the thing. There is no cure.

36

Born with AIDS

The newest and perhaps largest group to be infected with the AIDS virus are children born of drug-addicted mothers. Currently, one in sixty babies is born with the AIDS virus. Their mothers are often unable to care for them because of their own emotional problems or the child's physical problems. More and more AIDS babies are being fostered out.

Jane relates the story of Baby J who, for over a year, was like a foster child to nurses in a large eastern children's hospital.

Baby J was diagnosed with congenital AIDS at six months. She entered the hospital soon after being diagnosed, and she remained here until she died, some eighteen months later.

Her parents were I.V. drug users with their own physical and dependency problems, and they were unable to care for their daughter. Baby J also had a four-month-old sister who was removed from the parents' care. For about two months, she was placed in a hospital while she waited for foster care. Then she, too, was gone.

J had severe lung problems which required hospitalization. She needed oxygen most of the time. She'd just clear up from a lung infection and she'd develop another infection because she was so debilitated. It was a constant cycle.

Her chronic infections prevented her from thriving as a normal baby would. In general, her weight and development were very delayed. She did eventually walk. Her nurses bought her an infant walker and she'd scoot around in that when she was able.

Being isolated from the outside and her family was hard for this little baby. Because of their socioeconomic background, her parents didn't have their acts together. When the parents were drug-free, they'd be very solicitous to J, and they'd come to see her every day, but then there were long periods when they'd be back on drugs and wouldn't show up. So certain nurses became her foster moms, so to speak. They were the ones who cared for her throughout this year and a half.

The parents were very remorseful but, for whatever reason, they couldn't stop their behavior. Initially, the nurses and parents had no rapport. It's easy to say, "Be understanding and nonjudgmental," but when you grow attached to a little child and see her suffer, you can't always be empathetic to those who caused the problem. I think, as they got to know the parents better, the nurses' negative feelings changed. After a while, the parents felt comfortable calling up the child's primary nurse. If it was anyone else, the parents wouldn't speak with her. Eventually, the parents and nurses grew close. Even after J died, the nurses and parents continued to call each other.

Actually, the Gay Men's Crisis Group took over a supportive role for this family. Neither parent was gay, but the group felt a need to reach out to all families with AIDS. The parents were able to express their fears and anxieties with these people. The gay men also came in and spent time with J.

Several nurses—especially those who were pregnant—refused to care for J. The hardest group of people to deal with were some of the ancillary staff, such as people from housekeeping. They were afraid of getting the disease by emptying the garbage or that sort of thing. It was really a matter of education—once they got to know her, they just became very careful.

The nurses who did care for J volunteered to do so. They

had no concerns about acquiring the disease. You'd work on the unit and see them hugging and kissing her like any normal baby.

The hardest thing for them to deal with was knowing that no one had the legal authority to speak up for the child. By the time the child was close to death, the parents' involvement was minimal.

The child was assigned to the house staff, which rotated through the service, so there wasn't a consistent medical doctor in charge of J. There wasn't any communication with the parents on how the child's death would be handled—whether extraordinary means would be used to keep her alive. The staff nurses tried to speak up for the child, but they didn't have the power.

The staff didn't want any heroic measures used, such as a respirator, if J stopped breathing. They wanted her to be made comfortable. The day she stopped breathing, two house staff physicians found her. Because there was no order not to, they were forced to institute CPR. The family was notified and made a decision not to use extraordinary means. However, she'd already been intubated and placed on a respirator, so you couldn't take her off. She had a reaction to the medication, which was given in a vein in her leg. If she had lived, there was a high possibility that she'd have lost the leg. She died two days later.

It was tough for the nursing staff. They felt the child had been violated for no good reason, and they were angry. The staff was angry at the system for a very long time. I guess the nursing staff didn't see themselves having the power to intervene. Maybe they were also denying that the child would eventually die and then, when it happened, they wanted things to be changed.

The family came and camped out at the hospital. By that time, the primary nurses had a good rapport with the parents and felt a commitment to support them through this ordeal. Some of the primary nurses came in on their days off, and they set up a schedule that had one of them always there with the parents.

The loss of the child was very devastating to her primary nurses. They mourned this child as if she were their own.

There was a memorial service, which helped the nurses who were able to attend. Still, you don't get bereavement days when your patients die, and one of the nurses called in the day after the child died—she just couldn't make it in. We covered for her.

The clinical nurse specialist in child psych met with the nurses periodically to help them work through their grief. The primary nurses continued to support each other; they called each other and went out together.

It's been almost three years now. They've dealt with their grief somewhat, but even today, they still talk about J and what she meant to them.

PART NINE

CAREER CASUALTIES

The competitive health care scene today appears to work at cross purposes with quality caring in many of the situations the nurses in this book describe.

Nurses' endeavor to attain professional status through advanced education will be ineffectual until society and nurses acknowledge the nurses' right to care as clearly as it acknowledges the physicians' right to cure. Nurses' gender, ideology, history, and position as employees of institutions make it difficult for them to gain such recognition.

In this section, we hear the voices of discontent. They echo complaints vocalized by others in this book, but unlike the other nurses we've heard from, these nurses walked a fault line that split the ground under them and tore apart the careers for which they've worked so diligently.

37

Disenchanted

In a Manhattan apartment within a short walking distance of a renowned medical center, Beth's daughters, ages six and seven, play in their bedroom while we talk. Until now, Beth has chosen to stay home and raise her children. Their father, an attorney in private practice, works long hours. However, rising expenses are compelling her to consider entering the job market again. Beth graduated Phi Beta Kappa from Cornell University and entered one of the few two-year nursing programs that confers a master of science in nursing without first requiring a baccalaureate degree in nursing.

I left nursing to have my first child. That was eight years ago. I assumed I'd probably want to go back, but I've found, as the years have gone by, that I keep thinking of reasons not to go back into nursing. I finally realized that I don't want to do it. I *definitely* don't want to go back into hospital nursing, where I wasn't free to nurse.

I worked at university hospitals for four-and-a-half years on a medical unit. I started as a staff nurse and ended up an assistant head nurse. I had the opportunity to become a head nurse during that time. I refused, because I didn't want to take on that responsibility.

I don't see the kind of hospital nursing I did as being compatible with an active family life. I was going to the hospital at seven-thirty in the morning. The shift was from eight to four. The earliest I would get home was five, and often I would be there until six. It was almost an eleven-hour day. I rarely had coffee breaks, and I almost never took time for lunch. It was exhausting. Also, I never really felt that I'd completed what I needed to do each day, whether it was the physical care, the patient teaching, making care plans, or developing the admission interview which I was supposed to do.

I've had a recurring nightmare from the time I started nursing. It was four P.M. and I hadn't gotten out the morning meds, or there was something essential that I was supposed to do for a patient that I hadn't gotten around to doing. What was going to happen now?

If I had to do it over again, I probably wouldn't go into nursing. One of the reasons I went into nursing had to do with the age in which I grew up. I graduated from college, with a bachelor's degree in anthropology, during the Vietnam War. I felt I should contribute something to people, and I wanted to have a definite skill to offer them. I turned to the nursing profession. As a senior in college, it seemed like the perfect thing to do. The master's program I entered had a lot of people like me—people who'd been in the Peace Corps, teachers, and people who had been in other fields. We all were very motivated; we had what it took to get college degrees.

Nursing school just didn't prepare me for what would happen when I graduated. Suddenly, I was on the floor, being told what to do by medical students and interns with whom I had been in college. I was educated to be professional, just as they were, yet all of a sudden I was a "nothing." It was very hard on me. I'm a person with an ego, and I'm also a feminist.

The big concern of the doctors on the floor was whether I had followed their orders to the letter, or if I'd done some minor thing like find them a 20cc syringe. I really didn't like being told what to do, although I was at a hospital where the nursing department didn't expect us to wait on doctors. I knew that if I decided to buck the medical establishment in the best interest of my patients, I would have the support of the nursing administration behind me. I never was let down by nursing. If a doctor said, "I'm going to report you to your supervisor," I'd say, "Well, let me get her number for you." If they wanted to go all the way to the top, I would be completely supported in what I had done.

Surgeons always had trouble coming to our medical floor. They were used to the surgery floor nurses jumping at their beck and call, and we would not. They would threaten to report us for something as simple as not responding to a demand such as, "Nurse, get me that chart!" If I didn't like the way a doctor addressed me, I wouldn't do it. I wouldn't look up. I refused to acknowledge that he was talking to me. On our unit, we didn't jump when physicians said jump. The interns and residents soon learned that, but a lot of the attending physicians had trouble with it.

They also couldn't understand why, just because they had written something, we didn't necessarily have to do it. They felt that if they wrote an order, we had to carry it out. They didn't understand that nurses are responsible for their own actions. If something was wrong, or if something was not in the patients' best interests, we could refuse to follow an order, even when it involved treatment or a medication.

I remember a time when a female medical intern was called to check the unit of blood to be given. We never hung blood to be given intravenously to the patient unless both a nurse and doctor—together—checked the numbers and the written order for the patient. I called this intern to come up and do it. She insisted over the phone that I could do it by myself, that I didn't need her. I told her, "I'm sorry, but you do have to check this with me." I put the blood bag down and waited for her to come up.

Evidently, she came up in a big huff. She decided she was going to do it herself and didn't need a nurse to check it. She went to the specimen refrigerator where we keep stool cups, vomit and sputum specimens—the dirtiest place in the whole unit. She took an old bag of blood that had been used and was going back down to the lab. She hung it on this patient. When what she had done was discovered, she claimed it was my fault. She said I had refused to check it with her.

Fortunately, I'd gone in to see the patient, found the contaminated blood hanging, and realized I hadn't been asked to check it. I read the label and discovered that it wasn't for patient use at all. The patient could have died from that contaminated blood if I hadn't gone in there. I don't think anything ever really happened to the intern as a result of this.

I had trouble with some patients' families. When I worked over a long period of time with patients, I became very involved with their families, and I grew very close to them. They saw me as an important part of their family member's care. But there were always the families that came in and regarded the nurse as a glorified maid or waitress. Their biggest concern would be how many chairs they had at their side of the room, as opposed to how many chairs were on the other patient's side of the room. When we didn't see this as our biggest concern, they would get very upset.

One time, the head of the School of Dentistry had his mother in the hospital, and he was going on and on about the chairs. He wanted to know why I hadn't taken care of that. Someone asked me if I knew who he was. I said I didn't, and when she told me, I said, "So?" It shouldn't matter—and it didn't matter to me—who was doing the yelling, when what he was yelling about was trivial.

Other families were wonderful. Even after the patient was discharged, I would hear from the families. One patient, an elderly woman, was with us for months. Somehow, I must have made my way into her address book, because when she died, her son called to let me know.

I was working during the controversy over how much to tell patients. Do you tell them they are dying? Do you discuss "code or no code" with them? Nurses weren't allowed to discuss these things with the patient. If the patient asked, "Am I dying?" or the family asked, "Is my mother going to die?" we were not allowed to tell them unless the doctor had already brought up the subject with the patient.

We had to pretend we didn't know. It was difficult when you knew the patient was going to die very soon, when you knew you wanted to get the family members there so they could say what they had to say. You couldn't do it, even though the nurse was the one the family had approached.

I did enjoy working with families, talking with patients about their medical problems, making old and very sick people comfortable. Because my educational background wasn't confined narrowly to nursing, I was able to come into a situation and see all that had to be done for a patient. I always felt that we were never finished.

I also got along well with the nurses' aides and L.P.N.s because they knew I would never ask them to do anything I didn't do myself. Even when I was in charge of the floor, I was never holed up in the nurses' office. If I was finished with my work, I was always out on the floor, helping other people with their work.

Departments would refuse to do anything out of their realm, and then nursing would have to take up the slack. We moved beds. We went down to get food trays when patients were admitted after the dietary section closed. We transported patients to X-ray when no one else was available. We had a lot of R.N.'s in comparison to the number of aides. Very often, if the aide was overworked, we would do bedmaking. Sometimes it made sense to make beds, because you could talk to the patient while you were doing it, but we made a lot of beds with no patients to be seen. Even head nurses were doing things like moving beds, if patients wanted their beds by the window. Housekeeping help would refuse to do it!

Staff nurses work two out of three weekends. Since these are young women, there goes your social life. Two out of three weekends and a month of nights or evenings every other month was grueling. Because I was assistant head nurse, I didn't rotate shifts, and I only had to work every other weekend. This was the big luxury. How could I have worked all those weekends, when that was the only time I could be with my family? And how could you say, "I have to go home because my children's bus is coming"? I don't remember anyone ever just getting up and leaving. Maybe they did on some units, but not on medical units.

Sometimes, on the day shift, we wouldn't get to our charting until the evening shift started. You finally had evening people to take over the physical care of patients while you could start charting for ten patients at four P.M. That's why we would end up being there until five or six. There was no paid overtime.

Weekend staffing at times was very low. There would be weekends where I'd have seventeen patients and only myself and one aide. That would include a four-bed special care unit which had patients who needed intensive care unit-type attention. They needed oxygen and suctioning and nasogastric tubes and Foley catheters because they were completely paralyzed. If someone died, the nurse always took care of the body. If a patient went bad, the nurse had to stay at the bedside and the care of the other sixteen patients was left to the aides. I really worried about that, whenever it happened.

Some nurses seemed to manage to get in their cigarettes, take their coffee breaks, or take an hour for lunch. But then, there were a whole bunch of us who never sat down during the entire day. There was always something to be done in a patient's room.

I don't think I will be going back into nursing again. Although I met my husband that way, it's a hard job, even in New York, where people are reconciled to feminism. Nursing is a hard job if you have a strong ego. People assume that if you're a nurse, you're doing it because you couldn't be a doctor, or because you weren't good enough to do something else. It's hard for people to conceive of women or men *choosing* nursing over medicine, as I did.

I knew I didn't want to be a doctor. I didn't want to do what the doctors do on the floor. Yet it still hurts to have people think I wasn't capable of it.

My contemporaries—the people I socialize with—are primarily lawyers and MBAs. Nursing is sort of unheard of within the particular strata of people I deal with in New York City. There are a few social workers, because social workers don't get their hands dirty. That profession has a little more status. In New York City, you are what you do. It's not who you are, who you know, or what you were born into that's considered. New York is kind of classless that way.

I know there are ways to move up within the nursing profession, but I went in for direct involvement with patients, and if I'm not doing that, I may as well choose something else entirely.

When people ask what I do, I can say, "I'm staying home with my children," which is way down there in status. Few people I know in New York City stay home to take of their children. Or I can say, "I'm a nurse," which is also very low in status. I just prefer not to say what I do.

38

Squeezed Out

A nurse practitioner with a master's degree, Kathy has had a difficult time marketing her skills to a cost-conscious health community. As she tells us her story, it soon becomes obvious that her frustration is directed toward a system *rather than nursing itself.*

I'll tell you why I *think* I went into nursing: I am a product of the fifties, and nursing seemed to be the only occupation open to me. I came from a moralistic Baptist background, and my mother was a nurse. When the high school guidance counselor asked me what I wanted to be, I told her, "I guess I want to be a nurse."

She gave me nothing but positive reinforcement. She had no idea if I could hack the course work. She never once checked my scholastic record for my aptitude in science. I'd had teenage jobs in health care, and in the small mountain community in which I grew up, I only saw the bright women working as dieticians, social workers, teachers, or nurses. I also was very conscious of needing job security. My father had been unable to work for many years, and I wanted security for the future. It was only by accident that I obtained a baccalaureate degree and the liberal arts education, which opened up my whole world. I had mentors on the faculty who had a vision of nursing that I'd never considered possible.

My decision to enter graduate school came when I was about twenty-eight. I was just plain tired of being a nurse administrator. I was tired of continually coping with inadequate staffing and hospital administrators who didn't really understand or care what nursing was. Back in the early seventies, we nurses didn't know how to measure the care we gave, so we couldn't explain why we needed the staff we asked for.

One day, I told one of my favorite physicians on the floor that I was thinking of going back to school to get a master's degree in nursing. He closed the door to my office, sat down, and became very serious. Giving my hand a fatherly pat, he said, "Look, you don't want to be just a nurse. Let me send you to medical school." He never did understand why I preferred to continue in nursing.

It wasn't until the mid-seventies that my family life was such that I could become a serious full-time student again. The graduate education program I chose prepared me to function as a primary care nurse practitioner in joint practice with physicians. I saw that being a nurse practitioner was a way to remain in client contact, with good pay and autonomy.

I see the nurse practitioner role as much more complex than a physician's role. The physician obtains historical data of the ailment, does a physical assessment, and tests the wisdom of his diagnosis. He compares the information within the bounds of medical knowledge; he prescribes treatment. With nurse practitioners, the more information we collect, the more potential alternatives we can find for the patient to use to relieve his symptoms. We uncover the risks in each alternative and we learn the client's potential strengths. The client is suffering from the symptoms, whether they have a physical or psychological cause. The trick is to find the cause and do something about the symptoms, keeping in mind the patient's lifestyle, strengths, and goals.

I think my tunnel vision of the nurse practitioner role prevented me from seeing the realities that lay ahead. At the time, there was no question in my mind that becoming a nurse practitioner was the right choice. I felt that ambulatory care was the wave of the future, and being a nurse practitioner would offer me the challenge I wanted. That's where the jobs were going to be.

I was denying what the nursing literature was saying. Nursing leaders were expressing real concern about nurses' expanded roles. I failed to acknowledge that there might be problems, that there was potential to misuse the role. I was denying that we were being used to fill in gaps in physician services caused by a poor distribution of physicians. Now that there is a glut of physicians, we have become expendable.

I don't know, either, why I denied the power of organized medicine to stamp out a movement. I denied their power to change job structures, to appropriate our nurse practitioner roles for themselves.

In complete fairness, I failed to take into account the possibility that there could be nurse practitioners who couldn't do the counseling, teaching, and preventive aspects of nursing. They really wanted to be physicians' assistants. They were so eager to latch on to medical tasks that they became mini-doctors.

I prepared myself in a movement that lost its momentum—and that's a real sad feeling. I can't find a physician in this town who will practice in a colleague relationship with me. I feel like a child, with all these toys and no place to play. I'm in a transitional phase, trying to figure out how I can use my knowledge and skills.

Right after I graduated. I entered practice with my spouse, who is a family practice physician. I was reluctant to do so, but the choice was between taking a seven-dollar-an-hour job in an acute care setting, and going into my husband's office, where I'd done some of my graduate school field work. In short, it was the only game in town.

In my mind now, the experience in my husband's office was so ideal that I wonder if I was really in touch with reality when I worked there. People could hardly stand it when he closed the practice for personal health reasons. We're still grieving over the loss of this practice.

Overall, the best validation of how effective I was as a primary nurse practitioner happened when the State of

Illinois decided to open up its Nurse Practice Act to review the legal functions of nursing. Nurses from all over the state had to hurriedly mount a campaign to see that educationally qualified nurses be allowed to practice nursing outside of the direct control of physicians.

In less than a week, I mobilized my own clients. I sent a letter to each one, asking them to write their legislators and request that nurse practitioners be allowed to continue in practice. I received over thirty letters and many phone calls in support of my practice. Many of my clients drove four hours to the legislative hearings to personally testify on my behalf.

Basically, this is what was in their letters—"She taught me about health, and about how to take care of myself and my children. She listens, but it's more than the act of listening. She takes my health into concern and has helped me to do something about it." They were able to articulate that catalytic effect beautifully.

The catalytic effect of nursing is so elusive. Sometimes, it's merely a matter of feeding back support to a client, giving him self-confidence in his decision. I recognized the family problems caused by sleep deprivation in mothers and small children as well as the overwhelming fatigue of chronic illness.

Some of my catalytic effects meant letting people make decisions about their own bodies. I'd tell them, "These are your risks. These are the things you can't do anything about. These are the things you can change if you do this or that. Do you want to do anything? If so, what can I help you with?" I got credit for helping when it was really my client who did the work. It wasn't the advice I gave. I didn't say, "You should do this or that"—the mechanical sort of thing. *They* decided what they were going to do with their bodies, with their health, with their lives.

People had a need to ventilate their anger or frustration at insurmountable situations. I supported them and earned their trust. I was then able to get them into psychotherapy if they needed it. I also received referrals from the psychologist when she recognized that I could be more effective in a given situation, such as weight reduction, if I had these referrals.

I was a catalyst for getting people to follow their medical regimes. That was one of my real strengths. Although I didn't diagnose complex medical problems, when the problem was diagnosed, I saw that clients didn't just get a prescription. They got written handouts explaining what the drug was and *why* it should be taken. I'd guarantee that the client would get back to me. I didn't just say, "Let me know." I'd say, "Phone me Wednesday." In their letters, they translated this into "Kathy cared." That's so crucial to the patient following a medical regimen. One letter said, "Though I failed in my weight reduction goals, it was okay. I know Kathy will still be there to help me do better next time . . ."

I guess I miss all this. My husband was quick to relinquish the nonmedical aspects of our practice. He was more than willing to acknowledge that he was not educationally prepared—nor did he have the desire—to deal with client adaptation, stress reduction, anticipatory guidance, and health risk reduction. To him, these were "dump jobs." That was one reason I was able to practice as a nurse colleague in this setting.

Secondly, he was enthusiastic about our joint practice because it was a very busy practice, and a lot of the primary care encountered in this type of practice could easily be turned over to me. Telephone demands of clients were very high. He was accustomed to answering medical questions and giving basic directions. He didn't have the time or interest to pursue the reasons why people didn't always comply with his directions. For him, they either did or they didn't.

Following the medical regimen is as important to health as the right diagnosis or the right treatment. Medical schools don't prepare doctors for dealing with the whole people, their complex systems of health beliefs, their family dynamics, and their learning requirements. With me there, my husband didn't have to know these things.

He was also very willing to relinquish client ownership. Not all physicians will do this. I had a readymade job. It didn't take people long to ask for me when they wanted a wellness exam, when they wanted to understand their bodies better.

Some clients were uncomfortable with me. They liked a paternalistic approach; they needed and wanted to be told what to do. They didn't want to make decisions—they wanted the doctor to do that. They only wanted to look at the physiological aspects of their problems. They didn't want to look at their stress or the effects of their family problems on their bodies. It was difficult for some of the older clients to see a nurse in any other role besides an assistant to the physician.

I was very good at picking up subtleties. One thirty-year-old woman came in with a black eye, lacerations around her ear, and bruises all over her face. Since it was flu season, the doctor was too busy to see her right away. Once we had admitted her, I checked her wounds. I asked her how she got them. She mumbled something about falling down the back stairs, but I noticed her lack of eye contact, her shaky hands, and her eyes welling with tears.

We treated the wound, cleaned her up, and ordered an X-ray for concussion. The doctor examined her. I said, "What do you think about the wounds?"

He said, "The X-ray is negative, the wound clean. There shouldn't be any problems."

I felt there was more to it than that. I sat down, took her hand, and said, "Tell me again how you got these injuries." Tears streamed down her face. She ended up describing a long history of spouse abuse. We checked the records. Right there, in black and white, it showed that the physician had treated her for four years. There had been seven encounters—all injuries, each with a different reason.

I told her that there was no reason for her to be living that way. I gave her the name of a women's group, told her where there was a shelter and who to contact. I assured her that all this was her decision. I told her that if she ever needed to talk in the future, she should call me. I gave her my card.

She never came back to have the sutures removed, nor did I hear from her. A year later, she came back for a PAP smear. She took that opportunity to thank me for what I'd done for her. She said she had taken my suggestions shortly after her visit the year before. She left her husband and went to a shelter. They were now back together, getting counseling.

The catalytic effect is helping to raise consciousness, opening up alternatives for consideration. Sometimes, people are so stressed that they don't see any alternatives.

I made home visits, too, to the elderly who were too sick to come to the office and who could not afford an ambulance. I would visit and work with the physician over the telephone. We had to lie and put the visit under his name in order to get reimbursed. I made home visits to patients who were hooked up to oxygen and unable to leave home.

The visiting nurses weren't as skilled in physical assessment as I was. When patients at home needed a thorough physical assessment, the Visiting Nurse Association (VNA) would call me. We would put our findings together with a home care plan. It was not duplicating. I gave a thorough physical assessment and they implemented the plan. It was billed as a low-price physician visit, yet the client really got much, much more. We saved the taxpayer countless dollars. We caught respiratory problems while there was still time, and we did something about them before they turned into pneumonia. We caught high blood pressures and early bedsores. I'd draw bloods, collect sputum specimens. As a nurse practitioner, I was a vital link in that client's health plan. The VNA and the physician were paid for; I could not be directly reimbursed.

Because of my advice, countless couples bought approved car seats before their babies ever were born. The birthing process terminated far differently because I told the couple how to ask for what they wanted. Fathers took an active part in child care because I offered an alternative to what they were accustomed to.

When kids got my physical exams, they knew why I listened to their hearts and what exercise could do to strengthen them. I'd explain good nutrition and show on the growth chart what should happen. They could see measurable quantifiable results in the growth curve when they ate more nutritious meals. They would volunteer changes they had made when they came for the next visit. They knew I expected to be informed.

The parents got involved. I gave them references on sexuality and showed them the importance of explaining body changes to their children. I took body changes out of the closet. If the parents wanted to teach their eleven-year-old themselves, I would teach the parents how to do that. You have no idea how important that was. Many parents aren't willing to hear that their children need sexual counseling, but there were many who did take referral advice from me. If we hadn't explained the self-responsibility issues of sexual behavior, there would have been more little babies running around our offices in a year or two.

During physical examinations, I would explain the clients' genitalia to them and assess their birth control needs. I would teach self-assessment and give clients mirrors to see their body parts. As a society, we have to learn to acknowledge that sexuality function is just as important as heart function. I did this with men as well as with women. I'd lose some men because they weren't comfortable with me. Our culture doesn't accept that, either.

I helped persons with chronic obesity and heart disease to alter their lifestyles. Although I was qualified to work under a medical protocol, the real challenge was looking at their lifestyles with them. When they did come to a decision to diet, quit smoking, or exercise more, I helped them set up plans to reach their goals, plans that were realistic and achievable for them. Or I would recommend a referral system that would ensure results. If they had a complex nutritional problem, I would refer them to a dietician. If they needed advocacy in the social system, I'd refer them to a social worker.

I didn't make a difference to my husband's hospital clients. I wasn't allowed to go in to see them. I'll never forget the two-line letter I received from a nurse colleague and administrator in the hospital when I applied for staff privileges—"We are in receipt of your application. We see no need for your services at this time."

I knew the nurse professionally, yet she never attempted

to discuss my application with me. She—and others like her—are so quick to categorize all nurse practitioners as physicians' assistants. I'll never forgive my colleague for that letter, although she didn't know what she didn't know. She failed to recognize what a strength the client would have had with both an in-house nurse and myself working together to provide comprehensive care.

I harbor a lot of deep-down resentment toward a health care system that wouldn't facilitate a person with my skills. The public could have a far better system than we have now.

It has been terribly hard to share these things with you—things I have not shared so completely before. I think it's helped to be able to express my sorrow.

Why did I go into nursing? I'm still trying to answer that question. Now, at the age of forty and not being able to practice in the fashion I was taught, I have to ask myself, "Do you want to remain a nurse?" The realities of the health care system conflict with what I'm able to do and how I'm equipped to function.

POSTSCRIPT: Kathy is now in law school.

PART TEN

TROUBLED AND HEALING

Nurses buy into the Florence Nightingale syndrome; out on the battlefields, work yourself into a frazzle, turn around and go back again the next day. They deny that they are vulnerable to addictive behaviors such as alcohol and drug abuse.

There is no place for health professionals under the influence of alcohol or addictive drugs where human life is at stake. The profession has the responsibility to monitor its members and protect the public. Responsibility extends to the members as persons in need of help. Licensing boards are now replacing previous punitive actions such as loss of licensure with treatment options. Now, reemployment occurs under a closely monitored system.

39

One Day at a Time

Sondra is in her late forties. You are immediately drawn to her shining brown eyes. Her warm smile makes you feel good. You would like to have her for your nurse.

It's ironic that we're talking today—I just finished the best and worst year of my life. It was just a year ago yesterday that I was at the depths of despair, on an alcoholic binge. When I look back on that black, fateful night, I hardly believe it happened to me. In fact, I really don't remember much of what happened at all.

I had been denying the fact that I was an alcoholic for a long time, which was ironic, really. Not only am I a nurse, but my husband is a recovering alcoholic. So I'd been through it all with him. In fact, that's partly what precipitated my blow-up. He had relapsed, was quite ill, and had been hospitalized. That sort of jolted me. I gave up drinking for about a week. Then I caught a really bad cold. One of my colleagues at work suggested I go home and have a few hot toddies to cure my cold. Of course, I didn't need any encouragement; it only gave me permission to do what I'd been wanting to do all along.

Nobody at work suspected that I was drinking. I never missed work and I seemed to function okay. I stopped at Bay Liquor on the way home that night and got a bottle of brandy and vermouth. When I got home, I took a Contac for the cold and mixed some Manhattans. Again, I know better than to mix cold medicines and liquor, but my judgment was somewhat impaired. Besides, I didn't really care. My husband was ill and hospitalized. Life was really dismal. I just didn't care. I guess I was almost suicidal, but I apparently had enough insight to grasp for help. I don't remember doing it, but somehow I managed to call the Women's Crisis Line. I don't even know how I got the number. Later, when I was sober, I found it, in big numbers, in my address book.

The crisis counselor that came to my house that night was a man. Can you imagine the state I was in? Here it was, two in the morning, and I was so out of it I let a stranger into my house. He talked to me for a long time, trying to get me to admit myself to an alcoholic unit. I still couldn't admit I was an alcoholic; I only saw myself as being depressed. Finally, at about four in the morning, the counselor said, "Look, I have to go to work this morning: if you don't go voluntarily, then I'll have to call the police." He thought I was suicidal. Perhaps I was. I don't remember any of it. I must have thought he was bluffing, because I still refused. Pretty soon, the police came. They called my brother in Iowa. Jim convinced me to go to the county psychiatric hospital with the police. By morning, I was sober and trying to put things together.

I found myself on the schizophrenic unit. I knew I didn't belong there and really got panicky. I resorted to a real "nursey" thing—I demanded to see my patient care plan! There wasn't any, so I used that as an excuse to sign myself out. A psychiatrist finally came to see me and said, "You can leave, but you have to agree to go into a treatment program." I still wasn't convinced. I was ready to agree to anything, however, just to get out of there.

Alcoholics Anonymous sums it up well—"Alcoholism is insidious and cunning." You use a lot of denial, and you think you can solve everything yourself. Before this happened, I thought I could handle everything myself. I never confided in others. Now I have a "bitch" partner. When things get tough, I call her and say, "Let's go for coffee." I also have a sponsor through A.A., and I can call her, anytime, day or night. If I can't get her, I have a pocketful of other phone numbers—I'm never without them. If worse came to worst, I'd just go back to the alcoholic unit at the psychiatric hospital. In fact, the counselors urge you to use every means of support. Personal acceptance is something you don't always get outside A.A. or the alcoholic unit.

People have no tolerance or understanding of how this could happen to a nurse or doctor. They think you're weak. In fact, nurses and doctors think that alcoholism will never happen to them, and they can't tolerate it when it happens to their colleagues.

A recent article in the paper about alcohol- and drug-addicted nurses implied that nurses succumb because of the stress of their jobs. Frankly, I disagree. Sure, stress exaggerates any condition. However, everyone is stressed. If you, for whatever reason, are predisposed to be an alcoholic, you have to be extra careful. The stress is no different for nurses than it is for anyone else—say, for lawyers. You just need to find less self-destructive ways to deal with it.

Nurses reacted to that newspaper article. All who wrote to the editor took exception to the idea that nurses would have any human failings. They ignored what's right under their feet! One wrote that she had been in nursing for twenty-seven years and had never known a drug addict or alcoholic physician or nurse. How deluded they are! A professional who is in A.A. with me works with this nurse daily.

Those nurses' responses are really a reflection of the general attitude of society, "Those other people are the weak"—meaning the alcoholics, and drug addicts—"and we are the strong." It's even worse, though, when health professionals take that attitude. They're the ones who are supposed to be helping people like us. That's one of the reasons I don't blab to everyone that I'm an alcoholic. The director of nursing and a few of my key staff know.

As I said, this was one of the worst years of my life. Besides all I've told you about, my husband was diagnosed as having cancer of the mouth and is now being treated. We take one day at a time. It was the best year, because it's the first time in years that I've felt so good, so free. I never realized how the alcohol had consumed me, how bad I felt. I'd sleep eight or ten hours a night, but I never felt rested.

Now, mornings are great. I feel rested. I look younger. I have more energy than I've had in years. I've gotten a stronger belief in a Higher Being. I'm not embarrassed to rely on others, either. We all need each other. Patients need doctors and nurses, but doctors and nurses need someone, too. We sometimes forget that.

40

To Hell and Back

Claire's countenance shows little of the pain she has suffered for so long. She now seems at peace with herself.

Being a nurse, with the so-called stress involved in nursing, was not the cause of my addiction. In fact, it was the opposite. I don't know how I could have pulled through it all if I hadn't had my nursing to fall back on. For a long time, it was the only sustaining thing in my life.

Where do I begin? My story goes back a long way. I had a teenage pregnancy. My parents asked if I wanted to finish high school. The question itself was a shock. Just because I had made one mistake—the pregnancy—I wasn't going to make another. Of course I wanted to finish high school. I wanted to go on to college.

I had worked as a nurses' aide and I'd liked working with patients. I decided nursing was a good life for me. I'd always have a job, and I'd like what I was doing. While at school, I was surprised to find that I was truly blessed. I did well in school, and I really liked the classes and clinical work.

I attended a two-year nursing program. I was fortunate to meet excellent role models in my first job. They encouraged me to get more schooling. I decided to enroll in a four-year program, and I started working toward my degree. At the same time, I met and fell in love with a doctor.

We lived together and, eventually, married. He was good to my child. Later on we had a child together.

Then, he decided to move his practice to New York. He never consulted me and I never questioned his right to make the decision independently. I just moved with him. Here was my career, on the upswing, and I had only a bit of school left, and I packed up and moved, just like that.

Our new environment was a real cultural and value shock for me. I'd come from a small town and, even though I'd worked in a large city, I was not prepared for such a hyped-up scene. We lived near a university. The people and the health system were different. People seemed less satisfied with their lives. There was a lot of what I'd call militant behavior, such as nurses striking for their rights.

My husband worked long hours and did what many of the other physicians were doing to keep going. The erratic work schedule and long hours caused insomnia, so he'd take sleeping pills. Then, when he awoke, he'd be groggy and need a stimulant to keep him going. I can't believe it now, but at the time I didn't see anything wrong with his drug abuse. This was partially due to my rationalization and partially due to the fact that it was common practice—much more than people want to admit.

I didn't exactly like what the pills were doing to him, but I never even thought that addiction might occur. Besides, I was too unhappy to care. I didn't want to know. Our marriage was in trouble and, toward the end of it, I myself was taking uppers and downers. I was in pain, my marriage was ending. I used drugs to kill the emotional pain, and I was unwilling to face the fact that I could become addicted. I continued to deny that reality for several years.

As part of the divorce settlement, I was given full custody of our child but couldn't take him out of the state. I couldn't leave without leaving my child behind, so I stayed. For me, that was as good as a death sentence. I had no support system. I had no family nearby. I didn't do well in reaching out and making new friends. I was lonely, afraid, and generally not coping well.

I quickly got into another relationship with a man who was going to save me. I realize now that, while I had progressed in my professional career, I was still a child emotionally, always seeking out a parental figure in my relationships.

The man I dated was also a physician. He was the first to introduce me to cocaine. The first time I tried it, I thought I'd died and gone to heaven. It was the best thing since curly hair. It was wonderful. It really boosted my ego. When I took it, I felt like I could tackle anything. I remember taking some before a job interview. I went to the interview so self-confident and I sold myself so well that I got the job over several better-qualified candidates. Without the cocaine, I would never have had the nerve to go to the interview in the first place. Of course, a few months later, they realized I wasn't qualified, and they probably knew that I was on something, too.

I knew, in an intellectual sense, that taking drugs was not the right thing to do, but I rationalized my behavior. I gathered proof that it was okay. After all, two doctors—my ex-husband and my physician boyfriend—had used drugs, so I should be able to handle cocaine without problems. I talked myself into continuing my habit. There was no way I was going to give it up. It took care of my emotional pain.

It sounds like a cheap novel, but cocaine consumed my life. I didn't buy groceries; I didn't pay the rent. In order to maintain my habit, I was spending hundreds of dollars a week on drugs. I got into a relationship with a wealthy man. By now, I'd lost my job and people were wondering how I was sustaining myself. I couldn't admit my relationship, so I lied and said I had come into an inheritance.

I didn't seek help to discontinue my habit but, due to my physical condition, I sought medical advice. I was down to eighty pounds. I was concerned that snorting cocaine would ruin my nasal septum. I'd heard stories about the way cocaine eats away at the septum. I consulted an ENT [ear, nose, and throat specialist] man who assured me that this wasn't happening, and if it were to do so, he said he could rebuild it—he'd done it for others. He never suggested counseling or trying to get off the drug. Again, he reinforced what I wanted to believe. I'm not indicting him

—I'm just telling you how I continued to manipulate and use information for my own ends.

I was also having heart palpitations, so I saw a cardiologist. The doctor was most empathetic. If I had been able to be truthful I'm sure the doctor would have encouraged me to seek more professional counseling. But, again, I hid information to suit my own ends. One becomes very devious and clever with addictions. There was still a part of me that liked what the drug was doing for me and was unwilling to give it up.

Because of my relationship with physicians, I could keep my habits going—not for cocaine, but for other things. Coming down from cocaine was horrible, so I would need sedatives. I'd tell the doctor that I was agitated, just so he'd order me something. That went on for a while. If I got Quaaludes, I could sell those on the street for cocaine.

Concerns for my physical well-being led me to seek out psychiatric help. I started seeing a psychiatrist. But my confrontation with the fact that I was an addict never happened. Again, I rationalized. I was going to tell other people about cocaine. I was going to write a paper on the terrible effects of the drug. But I was unable to do anything about its effects on me. It was so bizarre and unreal. I was so ill at the time that I didn't even know how to apply for food stamps.

About this time, I was introduced to alcohol. I was agitated and someone suggested I have a drink. I didn't drink because I didn't like the taste of it, but I forced myself. I ended up having four drinks that first night, and I felt good. I thought, "Ah ha, now I've found a way. Alcohol is socially acceptable, it makes you feel good, and it's legal, cheap, and accessible." Within three months, I was a full-blown alcoholic.

The crisis came when I had a grand mal seizure. My brother came to rescue me. My ex-husband agreed to allow my child to move with me for a few months, with the stipulation that I would bring him back.

I spent six months with my brother. I got a job in a hospital and, because of my previous experience, I was quickly promoted. I took care of a very ill lady. Her husband was extremely wealthy, and he asked me to nurse his wife at home. I left my child in the care of my brother. At first, I really was needed, and soon I became part of the family. After the patient had been rehabilitated, I continued to stay on, in sort of a glorified housekeeper capacity.

I was still into drugs. It was easy—you can get drugs if you ask around. I sent for my child—which was illegal—and I continued to live in a grandiose style.

Things got worse. I finally called my mother and asked if I could come back home. I asked if she'd get me into a treatment center. She wasn't so sure that would work, but I went home anyway. In my typical self-centered manner, I didn't think about her or my brother, I just needed to get *my* needs met.

I started drinking again. I knew that being drunk wasn't going to get me the help I needed, but I was afraid of going through withdrawal. I lay on the floor of my parents' family room in a state of semi-consciousness that whole weekend.

I was so ashamed and afraid I'd have another seizure that I immediately went to the yellow pages and looked for the first treatment center I could find. I knew that if I didn't do it then, I might never do it. I called a center and they immediately admitted me.

At first, I only admitted to being an alcoholic. I was afraid to admit to taking drugs because they were illegal. I was also afraid someone would turn me in and I'd lose my license. Nursing was still very important and I couldn't afford to have that happen.

The staff was obviously aware that something else was my problem; they could tell just by the way I withdrew from the alcohol. I stayed at the treatment center for several months, as I was a lot sicker than I realized. At discharge, it was recommended that I go to a halfway house. I finally admitted my drug habit when I realized that no one would turn me in, that they would help me, that confidentiality would be maintained.

I returned to work under supervision. My urines were assayed for drugs, and I received counseling three times a week. I joined Alcoholics Anonymous.

Returning to work was a fairly easy transition. I was

fortunate to be hired in a hospital where the director of nursing was very open to helping recovering chemically dependent professionals. Initially, I worked with a head nurse who knew my history and verbalized acceptance, but sometimes she sort of had the attitude that she was holding this over me. I transferred and worked with two wonderful nursing supervisors. I did really well. They offered me a promotion and a transfer to another unit. At first I was hesitant, since I didn't know if I'd done well because of my work or if the transfer was because my supervisors thought so highly of me as a person. But my new supervisor gave me the highest marks on my evaluation, so I knew it was my work.

What helped me most? Before this, I never saw myself as religious. I counted on others, particularly men, to bail me out, but that didn't work. I believe in a Higher Being now, and I use that support. I also have my friends and partners in A.A. I now belong to several organizations that help nurses get off drugs.

I do some in-service for hospital nurses on substance abuse, but I don't tell them my story. I don't need that abuse. Their first reaction is that you are immoral. It's ironic—these are the same people who might take a Seconal from a patient's medication supply because they've been on nights and can't sleep. They never think this is wrong or that they'll get hooked. Their actions are moral according to their standards. We have a long way to go before health professionals see substance abuse—in themselves or patients—as a disease.

Several State Board of Nursing's reporting mechanisms even carry some degree of moral overtone. Those states put out a periodic written report that lists the names of alcoholics and drug addicts in the health professions. They don't list other diseases of professionals. I appreciate the concern for patient safety and concern that drugs are being diverted from patients. However, the majority of people I know, people who have been alcoholics or drug addicts, controlled their habits when at work. Diverting patient drugs is not as common as you'd think. It happens, but most of the time the nurses use outside contacts to get their drugs.

I personally diverted drugs—Percodan—only for a brief period, when I had no supply contacts. As soon as I'd made my contacts, I went outside the hospital, even if it was more difficult and expensive. If you take them from the hospital, you are afraid of being caught. Nobody wants to hurt patients, so you only divert drugs when you are hurting so bad yourself that you steal them as a last resort.

I don't want this to sound like a sob story. I just want to tell it like it is. Everyone is thinking all health professionals who are drug addicts are taking drugs from patients who are dying of cancer. That just isn't true, and it causes unnecessary anxiety for the public.

In some ways, this is the best time of my life. I have a very rewarding job in nursing. My still-constant pain and regret is that I no longer have custody of my child. It has been a big price to pay.

41

One of the Healers

Nancy, in her late thirties and pregnant with her third child, is in graduate school, working on her master's degree. She works part time as a consultant to a program for impaired nurse professionals.

Until recently, I coordinated a treatment program for professionals with addictions. All types of professionals were enrolled in the program—doctors, nurses, lawyers, teachers, and so on. Due to my pregnancy and school, I've cut back and now act only as a consultant and liaison between the State Board of Nursing and the local nurses' association. I'm helping to establish a peer assistance program for chemically dependent nurses. The program offers assistance and monitoring of chemically dependent nurses. It's intended to take the place of formal disciplinary action. There are probably about twenty-eight or so of these groups around the country.

Most of my professional career has been devoted to working with chemically dependent clients. People think it's odd for me to have an interest in this area. Many of the people who work with the chemically dependent are recovering themselves or have a dependent family member. Not so with me. I just enjoy working with these people. To me, alcohol and drug addiction are diseases. I have no feeling that those who are chemically dependent are immoral. My challenge is trying to lick these very devastating diseases.

Actually, drug and alcohol addictions are greater killers than cancer. Like cancer, they are out of the patient's control. But society doesn't see it that way. The prevailing attitude says the addicted are weak and deserving of no pity.

Society thinks it's the person's fault, so he doesn't deserve our treatment efforts. People think all an addict needs is the will to stop drinking or popping drugs. I wish it were that easy. Most nurses and doctors have attitudes similar to society. In fact, they're more unforgiving of their own than the general public.

The American Medical Association recognized this as a problem long before nursing did. Physicians have a peer assistance program in every state. In 1982, the American Nurses Association established a task force on psychological dysfunctions and addictions, with the goal of identifying the profession's responsibility regarding impairment of nurse colleagues. From that task force came the publication *Addiction and Psychological Dysfunction: The Profession's Response to the Problem,* which talks about the ethical and moral responsibilities of colleagues to help nurses with addictions. It also gives direction on how to establish peer assistance programs.

It is an important document because it shows people that we recognize that nurses are vulnerable to the same addictions as others, and that we're not glossing over this crucial area. I think it tells society we want to be responsible for the people who are taking care of them. It also tells nurses that we care and understand their problems, and that we will help them.

Though figures are conflicting, we know there are at least forty thousand alcoholic nurses. There are probably more. However, the rate is no greater than it is in the general population. It's a different story with narcotic addiction—it's believed that the rate of narcotic addiction is thirty to one hundred times greater in health professionals —that is, doctors, nurses, and others—than in the general population. The example given is that the population of ten nursing schools and three medical schools is lost annually to chemical dependency. However, we have few facts about the real extent of the problem.

Nobody knows what causes these addictions among professionals. People like to say stress is the causative agent, but that's not true. Certainly nursing and health care have lots of stress, but so do other professions. We aren't seeing addiction in solely high-stress areas, such as intensive care. Recently, in fact, we're seeing more nurse addicts from nursing homes. It's believed that professionals take drugs because of two factors—easy accessibility and what we call "pharmacological optimism." That is, people see what drugs do for their patients, how they relieve pain and bring a feeling of well-being, so they take them to do the same for themselves. Though professionals are very aware that addiction may be a consequence of pharmacological optimism, they deny this. They think they're too smart to get hooked; they think they'll know when to stop.

Though stress isn't the cause, it can accentuate the problem. We caution recovering clients to minimize stress. As you can see, much more research needs to go into the whole area of alcohol and drug abuse. We've only touched the tip of the iceberg.

Chemically dependent nurses are discovered in different ways. One notices behavior changes. Maybe a nurse has mood swings, or maybe she's using lots of sick days, or maybe her charting is illegible, with the writing going off the page. If patients are complaining that their pain isn't alleviated by hypos, an alert colleague may start putting two and two together. Once a nurse is discovered, administration usually applies pressure for her to obtain treatment or lose her job. That's usually how I get a call as a liaison to the State Board of Nursing.

Some people mistakenly think I can get them a job, so they call me. I don't care how they get in touch with me; once they do, I can help them and get them into some type of treatment program. We monitor the nurse and try to make sure she is complying, staying off drugs. We also help her to psychologically be able to resist drugs. If a nurse is not complying and is continuing to take drugs, formal discipline results.

One nurse came to me after spending a night in the drunk tank of the police station. Administration had the police come to the employing institution, handcuff her, and forcibly take her to jail. It's interesting—they don't treat physicians that way.

Dr. Leclare Bisell, who has written about alcoholism and physicians suggests that the reason physicians go to all lengths to make sure their addicted colleagues are taken care of is to protect their image as professionals. It's possible that attitudes vary because physicians are still mostly men and nurses are still mostly women, and drunk males are looked at differently than drunk females. Maybe that's why men seek treatment more readily than women. They know they will be accepted more readily.

Going back to work depends upon the employer and how open it is. If it's a long-term employee who has made a real contribution, the administration may open its doors. Some employers want little to do with addicted employees, even though employees in a work setting are under supervision and must submit to urine screening for drugs for a minimum of two years after treatment for addiction. What happens after that is not always clear. Hopefully, they have learned to use support resources. That's why we set up this assistance program, to see that they have a continuous personal support system. We still have a long way to go.

PART ELEVEN

AS OTHERS SEE US

Sometimes, people can buy into their own rhetoric. In the case of nursing, the true test involves answering a number of important questions: Are nurses as caring as they perceive themselves to be? Do they make the difference in patient outcomes they say they do? Do they offer the quality of care, consistent with the highest standards that they aspire to reach? Do others see professional nurses as they see themselves?

The lives of the four people in this section have been greatly affected by their experiences with nurses. They have had time to consider the role of the nurse, as it applied to them directly, as opposed to how the role is perceived. A doctor talks about the value of nurses as researchers, and patients and relatives testify to the effect of nurses on them during their times of crisis.

42

A Patient's Assessment

George suffered a respiratory arrest subsequent to a severe respiratory infection. He relates the experience, the meaning it had for him, and the people who surrounded him during his ordeal.

I don't remember the details, but I passed out in the living room of my house. Thank heavens my wife reacted quickly and called the paramedics. They did emergency resuscitation and whisked me to the county hospital's emergency room.

The first thing I recall is awakening to an irritating tube in my throat and the sound of people swarming about me. Then, no more. Next, I awoke in the intensive care unit. I had machines connected to my chest, tubes in my arms, and a breathing tube in my mouth. I couldn't talk. I looked up and there was a nurse, right there. That was a very secure feeling.

The nurses worked ten-hour shifts, seven days in a row, so I had the same nurses for long periods of time during my stay in ICU. I felt especially safe having the same nurse care for me, because she could tell what I needed before I did. For instance, when I'd start to get short of breath, she'd be there before I called. I guess she could tell from watching the machines.

I liked them not only because they were right there, but also because I felt they cared about the patients and liked their work. Both the nurses and doctors were enthusiastic when I was progressing well. I recall a doctor saying, "You're the kind of patient we like to see in here—you're getting better and you're going to leave voluntarily." That made me feel better. I wasn't going out feet first.

It wasn't just me—they were good with all the patients. I remember a man that lay next to me, separated only by a curtain. He must have been semiconscious when they were trying to suction his mucus. He was fighting it. They never got impatient with him. They kept talking soothingly to him, trying to calm him down. He kept fighting them. They never got angry, though I think I would have, had I been in their place.

I realized how good the nurses were, especially in a technical sense, when I compared them to the nurses on the general floors. The ICU nurses were very competent in techniques such as drawing blood; they were in and out of the vein like a flash. The general floor nurses stuck me several times before they could get in. I imagine they didn't have the practice.

The nurses were caring. They did things I can remember nurses' aides doing years ago, when I was hospitalized, such as giving you baths and rubbing you down. I never felt they thought these were menial tasks. It sure felt good and soothing. What was especially helpful was the way they communicated with my family. On several occasions, my wife missed seeing the doctor, and when she called, the nurse would read her the doctor's report. We felt like the whole family was considered and informed.

What I didn't like about intensive care was the noise. At first, you'd be glad to hear the machines because you knew they were saving your life. Then when you were getting better, the noise became annoying and you couldn't sleep.

I also didn't like the way they answered the call button. Someone at the desk would answer you, probably to make a decision about how urgent your call was. I didn't like that.

I only called when I really needed something, and I expected someone to be there for me, not to have to explain my need to a ward clerk who would then decide if the nurse should come or not.

I'm not a demanding person, but I did expect to get help, and I did find that once my need was known, I got it. For example, I had a headache and they secured an order for medication for me. Another time, I had a cough and wanted some cough medicine; instead of waiting until the next day, when the doctor would be making his rounds, the nurse called and obtained an order for the cough medicine. I was pleased and surprised by their actions. I guess I expected the nurses to have less initiative, to feel less like countermanding the doctor's orders. Yes, I expected her to carry out the doctor's orders, but I also expected her to be able to determine something is wrong with me before the doctor would and get help for me. I guess I don't see a cough as being that serious, so I was impressed that the nurse would go out of her way to make me more comfortable, especially when they have so many really sick people to take care of.

I felt so secure in that hospital that when I was to be transferred for a cardiac catheterization, they left me there instead. Different people, both doctors and nurses, explained things to me. I always felt I knew what was going on. One time, the doctor explained the cardiac catheterization; another time, a nurse explained what would happen in a test that measured the flow of blood in your arteries.

The nurse was helpful during my cardiac catheterization. She sat at my side and forewarned me of what was coming next. She told me, "Pretty soon, you'll feel your heart getting very hot." No sooner had she said this than I had this warm feeling in my chest. I really would have been scared if I didn't know what to expect, especially when you have signed a consent form that makes you aware of the complications that might occur. I was glad to have the nurse there, reassuring me that what I was experiencing was to be expected.

When I look back on it, my experience in ICU seemed so perfect because everything was handled so professionally. Everyone was efficient, dressed in uniform, and generally seemed on top of it. That's what I expect of professionals.

43

A Daughter's Memories

In her late twenties, Fran is blond and perky. We talk in the cafeteria of a large metropolitan newspaper, where she is employed as a journalist. As she speaks, Fran grows intense. Her speech is short and clipped, reflecting the anger she still harbors.

My mother died in 1972. She was fifty-nine. The last year of her life was an excursion into hell for us all.

She had several illnesses before the one that took her life. During her twenties, she had tuberculosis and a lung collapsed. When she was in her forties, she had a mastectomy. About twelve years later, she developed skin cancer over the site of the mastectomy. This was on the side opposite the TB lung. A series of radiation treatments was given and the skin cancer disappeared. She subsequently developed problems with her breathing.

At first, the doctors told her she had asthma and was allergic to our dog. The skin tests came back negative. After they had exhausted all allergy ideas, they told her the problem was in her head, since there was no reason for her to have difficulty breathing. We suspected the radiation had caused some problems, but the doctors denied this; they swore up and down that radiation could not have such side effects.

She became progressively worse. The radiologist attributed her condition to the spread of cancer to her lungs. Actually, the autopsy confirmed that there was no spread of the cancer. What she had was damaged lung tissue and cardiomyopathy caused by excessive radiation.

The consultant physician, who was the head of chest therapy, acknowledged this. When he saw my mother, the first thing he asked was, "Has your mother had chemotherapy or radiation therapy in the last few months? Because that's what is causing her breathing problems."

The doctors subsequently surgically placed a tube in her trachea so she could breathe. She spent three months in the intensive care unit before she was able to be moved out. In fact, she was the longest resident of the ICU. Perhaps today she might be discharged to a nursing home, but at that time her condition was such that no nursing home would have taken her.

The only break she got during that year was from the nurses, particularly the intensive care nurses. With the exception of the head of chest therapy, the doctors were fumbling, uncaring, inept, and made mistakes they refused to admit. My mother had an allergy to several medications. This was flagged on her chart, but the physicians either didn't look or didn't see it. I'll admit that the charts were voluminous. On three separate occasions, doctors wrote orders for drugs that my mother was allergic to and the nurse intercepted the order. I know this because I was there and saw it happen. After residents would visit, the nurses seemed upset and would shake their heads. It was obvious that the nurses had little respect for them. The doctors never acted on the obvious symptoms. My mother would have a complaint, such as her legs being swollen, and the residents would acknowledge the complaint and do nothing. Nor would they inform the attending physician. The nurse would make sure my mother's doctor knew.

I saw the nurses as my allies. My mother's color would change, and I'd ask the doctor about it. I'd either get no response or he'd pooh-pooh it. The nurse frequently made the same observation, and she'd be right on the physician to order blood gases.

I remember a particular time when the nurses came to my mom's rescue. It was mid-August, and the air conditioning went on the fritz. It was muggy outside, and the increased heat intensified my mother's breathing difficulties. God only knows how she was breathing anyway.

She was in an intermediate care unit, so she could be moved. The nurses made sure she was the first patient to be moved to the one area that still had air conditioning. They pushed that big motorized bed by themselves. There were no doctors or orderlies around. They knew my mother would feel better, so they moved her. It's that kind of consideration that I remember.

My mother was very personable. People liked her. The nurses showed up on Christmas with little presents, such as her favorite jellies. They sat and read to her during their breaks. They even came to visit on their days off.

My dad and I couldn't be there all the time. I was in school, and my dad had to work. It relieved our minds, knowing that she was with people who cared for her as if she were their own mother. You don't know how it feels to see your mother so terribly sick and have to leave her to others' care.

My mother was at home during the last weeks of her illness. We had exhausted the insurance benefits, and my father was mortgaged to the hilt. I was still in school. I cared for my mother after school. Dad was working nights, and he attended to her during the day.

My room was across from Mother's. She was good about calling only when she needed help. I'd try to get some sleep, and when her trach got plugged up, she'd ring for help. Because of the breathing tube, she couldn't speak well without covering the tube, and calling was impossible. We fixed her up with a little china bell. She'd dingle it when she needed help. I can still hear that thing.

The one fly in the ointment was the visiting nurse service. The nurse was fine—it was the policies of the agency that didn't serve our needs. For several weeks, the visiting nurse came twice a week to take care of my mother. She'd change the tracheostomy tube and that kind of thing. The cost was twenty dollars a visit, or forty dollars a week.

After the insurance ran out, and with the debts my father had, there was no money to pay for the service. We weren't in a category to receive additional aid. The nurse said she felt terrible, but she could no longer come to the house. I remember my mother, who was very weak by now, finding enough energy to boost herself up on one elbow and, with her raspy voice, saying, "You mean, after I've given to charities since 1929, they are abandoning me now?" The nurse's hands were tied. She stopped coming.

We managed somehow. If you want to call it fortuitous, my mother died six weeks later.

The nurses went outside the bounds of policy for my mother. On the day she died, we brought her back into the hospital at nine in the morning. She was in severe pain. The nurse was unable to contact anyone for a pain medication order. I said to her, "My mother is in great pain."

She said, "You're right. She needs something. Order or no order, I'm giving her something." And she did.

The nurses called the sisters to see her, and they called the priest to give her last rites. My mother went into a coma and died at seven that night.

44

A New Mother's Crisis

Natalie is a forty-four-year-old mother of six children. She describes her experiences with her daughter, who was born with a heart problem.

Aaron, my husband, always wanted a lot of kids. I became pregnant shortly after we were married, and I had a miscarriage. Then, twenty-two months later, I had Cory. He was beautiful, the perfect baby boy—the kind you see in the Gerber ads. He died the morning after he was born. I tried again and lost another one. Then I had Cathy—at home, with a doctor in attendance. I'm really glad we did it that way, because we were in control at home. Cathy weighed five pounds, nine ounces. Everyone went home, and there I was, with the baby. I told Aaron, "This baby doesn't breathe right; it whistles when it breathes."

He said, "Nonsense, you're just wound up. The baby is fine."

But something was not right. I called the doctor in the morning. I caught him at breakfast and told him that the baby wasn't breathing right. He said, "You're just upset with the excitement and all." But I insisted. Finally, he said, "Natalie, if it will do any good, bring the baby over." So I took her over, this eight-hour baby.

He checked Cathy and said, "Oh my God, you're right! Her heart valves aren't closed." He immediately called the local hospital, but its neonatal units were full. So they rejected my baby because they had no space.

My doctor said, "Natalie, my hands are tied; it's hopeless." Well, Aaron couldn't accept that. He called a friend who was the dean of the state university medical school. By the time he got in touch with him, it was noon. Aaron told him, "Natalie has lost three babies. If she loses this one, she'll go out of her mind." The dean said he would get the police helicopter to come pick us up and take us to the university hospital. He called back an hour later and—get this!—told us that the police refused to release the state-owned helicopter because it was to be involved in an air show in five hours.

Meanwhile, at our local hospital, they were preparing to move the baby and they screwed up and broke the lifeline to the lungs. Right away, Aaron called an ambulance for the three-hour ride to the university. It was terribly inadequate. They weren't going to let me ride with the baby; we were to drive behind.

By this time, I was convinced that she was going to die. I said, "Who are you to take away my last hours with my daughter?" They let me go along in the ambulance, but I was supposed to ride in the front. Of course, I crawled over to the back as soon as we started. I had to be close to my baby.

Then the power went out. They had to use emergency power, and they were watching her with a flashlight. I couldn't believe it!

The second we got to the university hospital, three doctors and three nurses met the ambulance. They worked on the baby for twelve hours. They were exhausted. I asked them what Cathy's chances were of making it. They said, "She's got a one percent chance." When I heard that, I felt like giving up. I was sure she'd die. But they didn't give up. They worked on her without stopping. They included us in every step of the way.

It was horrifying to see all those tubes and blood going into our little baby. But the nurses helped us. They converted a corner of the lobby into a bedroom, closing it off with a screen. They never once pulled me apart from my baby. They put a rocking chair right next to her incubator so I could touch her, be with her, and hold her feet. The physical contact was what kept me together.

For three days, they worked feverishly to get her to breathe right. I can remember one nurse standing over the crib, complaining to the doctor that her menstrual cramps were so bad that her legs were throbbing. He told her, "Sorry, but that's going to have to wait."

The doctor stayed two-and-a-half days, straight through. He never went home. They finally turned off the machine dials to stop the noise of the alarms going off all the time. They were all superhuman.

They kept me right there. Cathy's color was blue-gray. We were included in everything. I could see the blood come out when the baby urinated. They never kept a secret. It was like their own child was drowning.

They pasted the baby's eyes closed to protect her cornea from drying out. She was encased in a ventilator; her head was shaved so they could put the I.V. needles in her scalp. They explained that they were risking damage to her lungs to save her brain.

I didn't want to leave—not even for meals. Every minute, I was filled with the terrible fear that she wouldn't be there when I got back. This went on, day and night, for seven days. Finally, I went home.

The next day, they called to say that she was going to make it. She was through the crisis. With all she'd been through, her weight had dropped to three pounds, three ounces.

The third week they took her off the respirator and took her out of intensive care. She weighed four pounds, two ounces when they discharged her for the three-hour trip home.

The nurses were so wonderful. The whole experience changed our lives. It was the first time in my life, since losing Baby Cory, that I felt the world was a good place to be. From the very beginning, I knew that if there was anything that could be done, they would do it.

Fifty kids must have died in the time that she was there. They got all kinds—kids beaten, or babies the mother was trying to abort and get rid of. I could see how the nurses would despair when they lost one, and how happy they were when one was getting better. There was no friction between them at all.

They always did everything they could for the family. The nurses were not clock-watchers. They would work, not realizing that it was three hours past their time to get off. Parents left there in peace, even when they lost their babies. They knew that they'd had the best care possible.

The nurses treated the whole family, not just the baby. You felt a part of the life struggle that went on. Before I went home, they taught me how to put a tube down the baby's throat if she stopped breathing.

I wish it had happened that way the first time I had a baby. It was so different from my first hospital experience. It changed us, it really did. It was profound the way it touched our lives, and it still does.

The worst things about hospitals are the way you have to continually fight the policies and procedures. That didn't happen with this experience. When I had our first baby, I had to give nine arguments for everything I wanted to do. That's why I had my last babies at home. I believed in the natural way to do things.

In my first experiences in hospitals, I had a lot of real fights with nurses who bullied me. I suppose it's because, in the hospital, they have so little authority that they have to compensate by being drill sergeants. I found that the more education the nurses had, the more comfortable they were with letting you do things differently. You were less likely to be bullied. The educated nurse is more understanding and less threatened by authority. If the nurse sympathizes and relates to the patient—is not threatening—the patient does better.

I have personal friends who are nurses, and I know they haven't been given enough responsibility. They can make the difference between success and failure. When they can relate to the patient and can touch him psychologically, healing can take place. Doctors and nurses should be like salt and pepper—they go together. The nurse and the doctor have to be equals, and there has to be a bond there.

The nurse who is helping now with my in-vitro pregnancy is wonderful. I'd trust her over any of my doctor's partners. Nurses can do anything doctors can do. Do you know, she is not allowed to scrub for the procedure in the doctors' scrub room? Yet, they all stand around while she puts her hand up and rotates my uterus to get the follicles positioned for the implantation. The old lines have to disappear.

Without a doctor's trust, nurses have been unnecessarily limited. The medical world hasn't changed enough. The old ways continue, on and on. In the hospital, the people who know the patient have to make the decisions; we can't let the ones making the money run things. Nurses are the only ones taking care of the *human* relationships. They should be given more freedom to do that.

45

A Neurosurgeon's Insights

Dr. George is one of those rare physicians who acquired a Ph.D. because of a profound interest in research. Although he is a neurosurgeon, his present work is confined to animal and clinical research on spinal cord trauma.

Our conversation takes place in a conference room of the biomedical laboratories on the upper floor of a rundown coastal city hospital building. It's the Christmas season, and the labs are deserted. The quiet is a strong contrast to the boiling activity of the hospital floors below.

Dr. George, clad in jeans and running shoes, leans back and lights his pipe. He has apparently given considerable thought to nursing, and he talks earnestly, without pausing.

I think there are many kinds of nursing—different levels of nursing. At the bottom of the ladder is what's more traditionally thought of as the nursing "role," the person who does the day-to-day, nitty-gritty details of hospital care, such as transferring patients, keeping them clean, changing their beds, giving medication, and so forth.

Somewhere in the middle strata are nurses who perceive their responsibility as taking care of the psychological needs, as well as the physical needs, of the patient.

At the very pinnacle are research nurses, who essentially work in areas doctors don't work in. I think the middle and top areas have a much higher impact on patient recovery than physicians normally think they do.

My own contact with nurses at all three levels began when I was an intern in general surgery. I felt very acutely the loss of nursing care when the city budget was very tight. During that year, they had only an LPN at night. That simply meant that I, as the intern, had to get the medications, hang up the I.V. bottles, clean up the patients when it was necessary, and do the many things a nurse does much better. I missed the nurse terribly, and I think as a result the patients suffered a great deal.

At the university hospital, where they didn't have a budgetary crisis like that, the nurses essentially practiced what I refer to as the middle rung of nursing care. They dealt aggressively with the patient, from the standpoint of everything except the medical, diagnostic, and therapeutic decisions. I think the patients did very well at that hospital. As a doctor, I was able to do my job—that is, spend time diagnosing and making therapeutic decisions.

I have to tell you about one other breed of nurses—the operating room nurses. They're great. Respect from an O.R. nurse meant more to me, as an intern, than many other things, because the nurses knew what was happening in the O.R. If an O.R. nurse thought you were a good doctor, it really meant something—much more than if another doctor thought you were a good doctor.

Likewise, I apply a very similar judgment to our surgical residents on the surgical unit here. I'm very impressed when a new resident comes on to a ward and a nurse respects him. What it tells me is that this resident takes very good care of the patients.

I don't care how bright he is, how great a resident sounds at rounds, how great his clinical notes are; if the nurses don't respect him, something is wrong, terribly wrong. I think it's very important to use that scale to judge doctors, because nurses see the patients from the viewpoint of how well they're doing. They look at the whole patient. They don't just look at test results, the X-rays, or whatever. If a nurse believes that a doctor is taking good care of a patient, or that the patient is getting well, that says much more than the X-rays or the lab tests do.

In the last four or five years, essentially all of my contacts have been with research nurses. My experiences were not only in having research nurses working with me in implementing research programs, but I have also been reviewing grants by research nurses at the National Institute of Health. I think research nurses bring an insight and an attention to research matters that we, as physicians and Ph.D. researchers, don't think about.

The area of great concern to me right now has to do with whether or not patients believe that they'll have some recovery from spinal cord injuries. I am progressively convinced that there is a large role played by what a patient hears, sees, or is told concerning his chances for recovery. I'm convinced that both physicians and nurses tell the patients things that either enhance or retard significantly their recovery.

One example is the vast discrepancy that occurs between patients with so-called *complete* spinal cord injury and those with *incomplete* spinal cord injury. The medical dogma now is that if you're incomplete—that is, if you have any preservation of sensation or any motor activity below the level of the lesion—you have a good chance for recovery. If you come in with a complete spinal cord injury, you will probably never recover anything. In fact, many patients are told they have *no* chance for recovery.

From animal studies, I know that this is not the case. Animals show gradations of injuries and recoveries. They don't show this large gap between complete and incomplete. It's of great concern to me that this gap may be artificially produced by the prognosis the patient hears within the hospital.

Now this is an area that doctors very seldom pay any attention to. Nurses are very sensitive to these areas. I find, for example, no difficulty at all in convincing a nurse that such a phenomenon exists, whereas most doctors simply deny it outright. I believe that it is really on the nursing level that a major change in what the patient believes can be implemented. Doctors do nothing for spinal cord injury patients now; it's just nursing care. Without the nurses, and without the doctors who realize how important nursing is, the patients would die.

I work with two nurse researchers. Doris Weber has a critical care nursing background and is now our coordinator for the spinal cord injury department. She administers our clinical double-blind randomized study. She is the person other hospitals contact if they have admitted a spinal cord injury patient. She keeps our research records on all patients. Finally, she is the person who organizes and arranges our testing protocol. I go to her whenever anything has to be done on any spinal cord injury patient, whether it involves giving a neurophysiological test, taking some central spinal fluid, or getting a record. I go to her for her insights into what's happening with a patient. Data analysis relies on her insights about the patient's clinical behavior quite a lot. When the tests tell us the patient should be able to do things he's not doing, I then go to Doris to get her insights into what other things are going on in the patient's head—things that are affecting his recovery.

The other nurse, Alice Carter, coordinates the Regional Spinal Cord Injury Center for the Institute of Rehabilitation. She, too, is essential to all of our work. Without Doris and Alice, the research at this medical center could not be done.

Because of my research interest in brain and spinal cord injuries, I am on the NIH committee that reviews clinical investigator development awards. On the average, I see one or two grant applications from nurses, three or four times a year. I have to admit that their applications differ sharply from the medical ones I read. They use language and behavior approaches that are totally different. They cite literature that I've never heard of. There are some marvelous ideas.

Unfortunately, I think institutional support for nursing research is very low. If you find any support at all, it almost always comes from the nursing school and very seldom from the medical school. I've looked at a number of grants from nurses who have very bright ideas. They talk about the psychological profiles of patients as well as all these methods for manipulating the social and psychological environments of patients. These are things that I don't know anything about. By the dint of her own enthusiasm, a nurse researcher may convince someone in the medical school, and the doctor with whom she works, to be very enthusiastic about her ideas.

However, medical school support has been so low that many of these nurses cannot and will not get the funding to do this kind of research. It's sad. I wish the situation would be different, and I wish that the nursing schools would be better integrated with the medical schools. There shouldn't be separate faculties for nurses and doctors. I think that combining them would go a long way toward essentially bridging the gaps in areas that I, as a doctor, know nothing about. My education never included anything about nursing.

There are enormous gaps in physicians' education. I think there are more gaps in physicians' education than there are in nurses' education. Nurses are required to know a lot of what doctors know. Nurses get the medical training, but doctors don't get the nursing education. It's unfortunate, but that's been the history of the dichotomy between medicine and nursing.

I don't think you can change the older doctors and nurses who have been in a very different environment. I think the real issue is to meld nursing schools and medicine schools, have medical students attend nursing classes. Only in that way will a medical student ever learn the language, the history, and the research that's going on in nursing. And there's a lot going on! When I look at a grant and it has two hundred references to things that I've never heard of —I wasn't even aware this kind of research was going on— it tells me of the gap I've had in my education.

I recently reviewed a grant prepared by a nurse who is interested in brain function. She's applying for a five-year clinical investigator award. She wants to carry out a study on brain tumor patients, to see if their brain functions correlate with their recovery from surgery. If the patient can sense his condition, will he recover from surgery more quickly?

The patients' perception or ability to perceive their condition is bound to have a large impact on recovery. Brain tumors have a profound effect on how the patient perceives his condition. If we're able to discover to what degree the patient understands his condition, then we can tailor therapies according to the patient's perception. This kind of research would be a major breakthrough in the care of brain tumor patients.

Unfortunately, the grant will probably not be awarded. One of the key criteria for grant awards is very strong institutional support. This nurse doesn't have it from her own colleagues in the nursing school. They won't guarantee a long-term appointment. They feel she is going into too medical a subject.

They're saying, "Well, we don't know what her future will be with us if she doesn't get her proposal funded. We've considered giving her a little bit of lab space." Currently, she's using lab space that was loaned to her as a favor from a physician. Frankly, I think her faculty colleagues are prejudiced because she was working so closely with a physician.

I would very much like to see both medicine and nursing, especially the neurosurgical department, support her research. I would like to have them say, "Our neurosurgical department has an investment in this nursing approach to neurosurgical care; therefore, we're going to contribute to that kind of investment."

I don't think it's going to change unless those things happen. It's very sad, because doctors have this blind spot —they don't deal with these sorts of things. Not only that, I don't think we are capable of it, nor should we deal with some of these things on a day-to-day basis. It's like when I was an intern and there were no nurses and the ward was in trouble. My training and my background were essentially in making diagnostic and therapeutic decisions and going into the O.R. When it came to making sure the patient was comfortable and getting good care outside the O.R., particularly in an instance such as a spinal cord injury, where the care is basically nursing care, I had no preparation.

In neurosurgery, spinal cord injury is a very unpopular area among neurosurgeons because they can't do anything. They can't operate. There is no drug for miraculous recovery. It's basically nursing care. So you find that most neurosurgeons avoid spinal cord injury patients. They go into things that they can cure in the operating room, situations where nursing has very little impact.

Or take the example of a patient with severe head trauma. What is required is nursing care, not medical care. There is nothing that physicians involved with a severe trauma case can do. But what happens to all these patients, whose diseases require primarily nursing care for recovery?

One of the most unfortunate things I see happening is that a lot of good people are leaving nursing. Some of the best nurses I know have left. We have this very good friend who was the head nurse on neurosurgery. She was great as a nurse, but she's now gone into law. I think it's a great loss to nursing. I've known a number of nurses who have gone on to become doctors. It's nice that they became doctors, but what's not so nice is that some of the best minds in nursing should be leaving nursing.

In a nutshell, I think nursing should be a specialty of medicine. It should not be a separate profession. There will always be certain diseases in which the treatment is nursing. There will always be a very, very large population for whom medicine can do nothing, because anytime a disease becomes curable, the proportion of patients with incurable diseases increases. After all, people have to die of something.

When you don't have the magic bullet, when you don't have the single operation or whatever, when the diagnosis is known, when the CAT scan has been done, over half of what's left is nursing.

EPILOGUE

A Nurse's View of Nursing

The office of the State Secretary of Licensing and Registration is elegantly furnished. Autographed portraits of famous nursing and political leaders adorn the walls. The scribbled phrases on the portraits express the high regard for the woman who works here. A framed poem also catches the eye. Its words speak of the power of persistence. Alongside is a calligraphic commendation from the National Black Nurses' Association.

It is here in her office that Marla considers her career—and that of the nurse of the future.

For me, nursing has been just a wonderful career choice. I've had such varied and rich experiences in nursing. I started doing staff nursing in Boston, working primarily in critical care. Then I joined the Navy and had the opportunity to see a totally different system of care delivery.

My first ten years in nursing were spent in direct care. During my Navy experience, I received a commendation of merit for giving good care to patients. Somewhere, though, early in my career, I focused on moving into management positions where I could impact a broader spectrum of people and situations. I wanted to be in a position that gave me breadth of operation.

In general, I see nursing from two perspectives. The first is a personal perspective based on my experiences as a former president of the American Nurses' Association. While I held that position, I traveled throughout the country and saw nurses in a variety of settings. What impressed me most were the numbers of bright, committed nurses working all too often in situations where resources were scarce. You discovered the ingenuity of nurses and their advocacy for patients. It was exhilarating to find compassion and caring still out there.

I recall going to meet with nurses in New York who, as representatives of thirteen hospitals, were working toward collective bargaining. They talked about not having necessities such as linens, soap, and bedpans. The hospital systems were designed for bulk ordering and the intensity of patient care was not considered when staffing. So supplies were always short and there was no managerial response to the nurses' verbalized concern for patients' welfare. From the nurses' standpoint, the system did not even provide the basic elements to take care of sick people.

When a system has fiscal problems, administrators deal with them by reducing staff. You may still have the same number of patients with the same needs, but management expects the nurses who are left to do more work for the same pay and with fewer resources. The nurses become stressed and this interferes with their ability to function. Staff nurses bargain to change these things.

The second perspective I have of nursing is of the nurses in our professional organization. I've found these nurses to be somewhat schizophrenic. On one level, they are bright, articulate, and do a very good job of presenting the membership with a contemporary definition of nursing, its practice, and its prowess. On the other hand, they tend to be myopic, rigid, stultified, and unable to understand that the structure of nursing in the future is contained in what we're doing in the present.

To me, the classic example of how this dilemma is manifested is in the "entry into professional practice" issue. The current disagreement among nurses focuses on whether professional nurses should have baccalaureate degrees as a minimum of preparation. By having nurses hold everything from diplomas to doctorates, we have no universal codification of our professional knowledge. That's a real dilemma when you're trying to compete in a health care field that's undergoing rapid transformation. You're competing in a market where other health providers have a much more unified and solid educational base.

The problem is the lack of understanding of the results of a given type of education. Higher education is essential to our practice; you can't do what you don't know. We can no longer fool ourselves. Right now, only about 35,000 nurses out of the 1.7 million total have master's degrees. As a profession trying to reach professional status, our educational mosaic is limiting.

Many nurses, regardless of whether they think nurses need a baccalaureate, seem fixed on titles and licensure. They wrangle over whether a two-year nurse should be called an associate nurse or a technical nurse. We need to remember that education brings more than a title; it brings knowledge that should make a difference in a health care system that needs innovative people who can think and make good decisions. If we're going to have practice that responds to a changing health care system, we must have a high level of education. Nurses are incorporating a wide array of technological advances into their practices, yet they fail to recognize these additions as an expanded base of knowledge. I find this an interesting paradox. Other than nursing, no profession in the health care system will settle for less than a baccalaureate preparation. Social work is talking about requiring a master's degree; so are physical therapy, occupational therapy, and dietetics. Pharmacy is talking about a clinical doctorate, while medicine is considering a move to a five-year curriculum because of the expanded knowledge base. In a marketplace that is becoming increasingly competitive, health professionals will be valued in accordance to their educational preparation.

We nurses expect to continue to be in charge of people and systems that affect our patients, but this is being challenged. When I was president of the American Nurses' Association, a bill was introduced in California by psychiatric technicians. These are individuals who work in mental health facilities. By law, their minimum preparation is a master's degree. They refused to take orders from nurses who had only hospital diplomas. They argued that their basic preparation and knowledge base was more advanced than the nurses', and therefore they should not be directed by the nurses. Health workers compete for turf rights.

Although this event was seen as an isolated case—and idiosyncratic, in terms of California—it's a signal to nurses that we need to look beyond our own navels. The problem with the issue of the baccalaureate is that, for many nurses who don't hold one, it's as if you were personally attacking them for a choice they made way back when. They take it personally.

The profession must think collectively. We need to form a coalition and identify the people who support us in the issue of entry into professional practice. We need people outside of nursing to support us—people like hospital administrators, directors of nursing, college administrators, physicians, and other groups who have used the legislative route to mandate the baccalaureate. It can't be just the nurses who support the baccalaureate versus the nurses who support fewer years of preparation.

The preparation needed to enter into practice is the major issue in nursing, not only because of the issue itself, but because our fixation on the issue saps our strength and keeps us from focusing on getting ready for the future. While nurses were upset and fixated on the issue of the baccalaureate degree, there were twenty groups last year that sought licensure from the state bureau. Some of their licensure acts could be said to overlap or prohibit what nurses do. Other groups aren't standing still while we work this out.

Take lay midwives, for example. We've had certified nurse midwives [CNMs] around for quite a while. So why, in the face of lay midwives emerging as a new aspect of health care, haven't nurse midwives been able to sell themselves as an option that is already in place? I ask the question, but I don't know the answer. See, throughout the debate over lay midwives, people were saying that certified nurse midwives were already here and they provide better service than a lay person could. What CNMs need to do now is go public with this argument and have the public argue for them. Again, the issue becomes political. You need other people to see you.

You learn strong observation skills when you work with the sick. As a psych nurse, I learned to keep process notes and write down things as I observed them. I use those same skills in my everyday work as state secretary. In my current position, I observe which legislators are talking to each other, which appear to be united, which are assigned on committees together. I observe if they share the same ideology. What does all this tell me, in terms of introducing ideas to them, deciding how to intervene, and seeing if it works? It's the same process we do in nursing—assess, intervene, and then evaluate if the intervention worked. It's fascinating.

I find that, in a political environment, things are cyclical and repetitive. When I review my notes, I find insights into how this group works, or how those people think. I discover connections between things I hadn't noticed in isolation—things you would not think relate—but they do.

The informal system is strong in the political environment. Personality is a major influence. You may or may not obtain resources, depending on how your personality fits with the one you're attempting to influence. You need to get to people before you bring your case to the legislature.

For example, people usually develop a memo, send a letter to all the legislators, do it two or three times, and feel the legislators are informed. I've found it more productive to decide on a few key people, seek them out, and really make them interested in the issue. Political relationships are all-important in getting one's point across. What you need is one highly influential legislator to hold on to your issue, like a dog with a bone, and you have it made. That's all it takes. One person can make—or stop—the whole show. This one-to-one process takes a lot of time, but it pays off.

We nurses have learned about the political process, but we still have a long way to go. We need to identify nurses who have educational and political savvy. We have to mobilize them and put them into important positions where they can move things along for nursing. So many times, there isn't the public support for nurses in nontraditional roles, such as nurses holding political office. We need nurses to be in the legislature as our spokespersons. We have several, but we need more.

Clearly, tomorrow's health care is going to be different, and nursing practice within that context will be different. Tomorrow's skills will be different from the skills that are needed today. I don't know what those skills will be, but we need to put a strong educational base in place now.

I've had the privilege of serving on the International Council of Nursing's Board of Directors, and I've certainly come to appreciate that nurses in the United States have the greatest knowledge base, are the best technologically, have the best professional organization, and receive the highest pay in the world. Still, women are leaving nursing, and current high school graduates aren't choosing nursing. We're not in competition with law, medicine, engineering, and other nontraditional occupations for women. The diehards are claiming that we're not attracting people because we're pushing the idea of baccalaureate preparation, but the statistics negate that idea. Women in droves are going to law school, which involves a much more lengthy and rigorous education. Rather than discouraging women, the baccalaureate for entry into the profession of nursing should attract them.

I can see that it's difficult for bright young women to choose a career in nursing today. There are a lot of archaic stereotypes about nurses. The contemporary woman is asking. "Why be a physician's handmaiden when there is no consensus on the education needed for the profession?" Few really know what the nursing career paths will end up being, and there is so much stress that results from that uncertainty.

Yet, I would advise my daughter, or anyone else, to go into nursing. I think it's a wonderful choice. It prepares you for life, living, and motherhood. You learn about your body and others' bodies, and you gain a whole level of knowledge that others don't have. It's good for you as a person.

Professionally, nurses have access to a variety of career pathways. You can be a clinician, an administrator, a researcher; you can teach if you so desire. Very few other professions have so many options.

What would I say my own contribution to nursing has been? That's an interesting question. I haven't thought of what my epitaph should say! I guess it would be that I worked to make nursing stronger as a profession.